LIFE REVISITED

Humbly dedicated to my wonderful parents, Barb and Noel, without whom this book would never have been possible. I am indebted to their unconditional love, tireless support, and remarkable characters, the likes of which I can only aspire to emulate in part.

And to Sia, for teaching me the true nature of love, showing to me that which is worth striving for in this world, and being an endless source of inspiration.

Life Revisited

Finding Meaning and Purpose in an Age of Nihilism

LUKE SCHILLER

Published in Ottawa, ON, Canada by IngramSpark[SM]
In association with SchillerAcademy[TM] (www.schilleracademy.com)

First Edition (Paperback) 2018
ISBN 978-1-9995082-0-3

LIFE REVISITED: FINDING MEANING AND PURPOSE IN AN AGE OF NIHILISM

Contents

The Schillerian Model of Meaning & Purpose

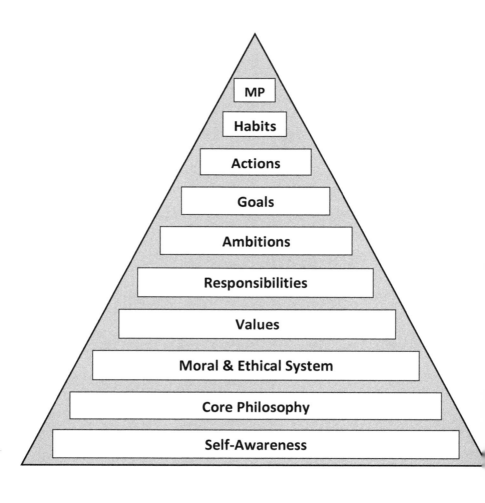

How to Use This Book

I'm going to be upfront with you from the outset – this is not a standard self-help book. I'm not here to spend 200 pages of your time dictating how you should live your life and what your central meaning and purpose is. Instead, I wish to provide you with the relevant knowledge, fascinating insight, and a practical framework for you to find the answers that you are seeking and to arrive at an understanding of your *own* sense of meaning. I'd like to help you achieve this through the careful creation of your very own **Foundational Document**, which will serve as an immensely valuable tool for navigating through this often puzzling journey called 'life'.

What in the world is a Foundational Document, you ask? Well, simply put, it's a fancy name for a document that details everything that is necessary to establish your own sense of meaning in life *and* how to act on it. Sounds tough, right? Don't worry – the process is surprisingly simple and operates in a helpful step-by-step manner. Here is how it works.

At the end of some of the chapters in this book, beginning with Chapter 3, there will be a few questions for you to answer in light of the new knowledge and insights you have acquired from those respective chapters. All you will have to do is write down the answers to those questions in whatever way is most convenient for you, whether that is on a laptop or using the classic (yet perhaps slightly outdated) notebook and pen/pencil method.

By the time you finish this book, you will have created your own Foundational Document that will outline exactly where you derive your sense of meaning from and what you are meant to do with your life as per your discoveries. The great thing is that you will always have this document to reflect upon, and I think you will find it to be extremely valuable as you progress through your life.

It is helpful to think of the process contained in this book as being akin to fitting puzzle pieces together. If you are trying to complete a puzzle and have not yet seen the picture that the pieces will make ahead of time, you don't necessarily understand what you are creating until the pieces begin to form a complete picture. However, from the outset you do know broadly what it is that you are striving for in the end (a complete picture of your life meaning and purpose, in this case), but you just do not know what it is *exactly* that the picture will show you.

The things that you will learn throughout this journey (both from the book itself and about your own self) will operate in a similar manner to gradually piecing a puzzle together. Striving to gain an understanding of your sense of meaning in life and your purpose is a gradual process that you must work towards if you are to be successful. As you proceed in this book, I think you will find that the puzzle pieces will start to 'click' and you will gain more and more clarity as you go along, culminating in a breakthrough in Chapter 8.

When perusing the available literature on the topics of meaning and purpose, I noticed a distinct binary nature in terms of the authors' approaches. Either the books were overly complex and academic in nature (such as a massive philosophical treatise the likes of which would probably just confuse people even more), or they were overly simplistic (i.e. 'just believe in my conception of god and you'll find meaning!')

Observing this problem assured me that I was making the right decision in writing this book. There appears to be a great need for a concise work on this otherwise complex topic that strikes a balance between being informative and being practical, and I would argue that it is needed now more than ever. Instead of confusing you or strictly telling you how you should live your life, instead I wish to provide you with valuable knowledge and a practical framework that helps you build up a sense of meaning and purpose that is not only relevant to you, but is *established* by you through the use of ground-breaking insights.

I am thoroughly convinced that by the end of this book you will have a vastly more consolidated vision of your purpose, just as so many of my clients have had even though they used a more primitive and less developed version of this method. With the additional knowledge that you gain from this book and the life framework that you will build in the process, I am positive that you will be immensely successful in finding meaning and purpose in your life.

So, in what form will these unique insights come? Here is a brief breakdown of what we are going to explore:

Introduction – In the introductory chapter of this book we are going to explore something which people are starting to become more aware of: a crisis of meaning that people all across the Western world appear to be undergoing at this very moment.

Chapter 1 – In order to understand your own meaning and purpose, it is imperative to understand how and where humans have found meaning and purpose throughout history. This chapter will allow you to see how meaning has traditionally been discovered and how the concept has changed over time for humanity as a whole.

Chapter 2 – After having learned about the trajectory that the concepts of meaning and purpose have taken throughout human history, we will be able to more accurately understand how exactly we have arrived at our current crisis of meaning. Understanding the *five major trends* that caused humanity's crisis will allow you to pinpoint where exactly your own unstable sense of meaning and/or purpose originates from at a more foundational level.

Chapter 3 – In Chapter 3 we will take a look at very interesting and useful conceptions of the terms "meaning" and "purpose" in order to provide guidelines that will help you define what these two terms mean to you on a personal level. In order to reach an understanding of your meaning and purpose, you must first know what it is exactly that you are looking for when you use these terms. Informed by the knowledge acquired from the previous chapters, this is where your own journey will truly begin.

Chapters 4 & 5 – These two chapters are all about self-discovery. Knowing the unconscious beliefs you hold, the things that have influenced you throughout your life, and your own conception of positive and negative events in your life will allow you to truly understand yourself and your capabilities. To understand thy purpose, you must first *know thyself* (The ancient Greek philosopher Socrates would be proud! He coined that maxim, after all.)

Chapter 6 – This chapter will assist you in establishing your own core philosophy, something which serves as a foundation for all meaning and purpose-related ideas. To truly understand and act upon your own meaning in life, you have to know where you stand with regard to the origins of life and existence in general.

Chapter 7 – In Chapter 7, we will work together to explore and uncover your own system of morality, which will have the effect of providing guidelines in your life that more clearly direct you toward fulfilling your developed purpose.

Chapter 8 – In Chapter 8, we will look toward the future at who you *will* be moving forward. This will be informed by the journey you will have taken so far as well as your values, responsibilities, and personal goals. We will create a roadmap for you that is informed by your true purpose and your conception of the meaning of life. Your journey in adhering to this roadmap will go hand-in-hand with fulfilling your purpose; the two are one and the same.

Without any further ado, let us examine why it seems that so many people are lacking direction in today's society; the symptoms are laid out in plain sight.

The Fractured States of Meaning and Purpose

Plainly speaking, we are living the in best period in human history. There is no other way around it. Among numerous other things, a higher percentage of the Earth's human population has access to a stable food/water supply, shelter, electricity, and an education than ever before. Worldwide rates of poverty and deadly disease are consistently declining at a rapid speed thanks to continued economic development and unparalleled medical access and advancements. With the exception of a slight rise since the events of 9/11, global deaths from war and conflict per year have been on a rather consistent decline since the end of the Vietnam War in 1975 and are at their lowest rates per capita since the late 1800s.[1]

Access to incredible technology such as the internet and smartphones is also becoming increasingly widespread, allowing for nearly instant communication across the planet and the unprecedented sharing of knowledge and information. There are more stores and services than ever before (many of which exist online within an electronic device in homes around the world), allowing for nearly instantaneous access to the purchase of products and services that make life easier and more comfortable. The availability of liveable occupations and the use of easily accessible tools for self-created opportunities in an open market is more extensive than ever before. These factors afford individuals with the opportunity to make meaningful contributions to their local community and their broader society with relative ease.

With the exception of looming threats such as climate change and political polarization, there is every good reason to be optimistic about the future of humanity and to continue working hard towards our increasing prosperity as a species. Never before has it been so good to be a human being, and yet a crisis is bubbling beneath the surface that is more prevalent among those who live in the more developed countries such as those found in the Western world, ironically enough. There appears to be a massive and widening discrepancy between our physical and mental/emotional prosperity, the likes of which I would argue has never been seen before on such a large scale.

This truly is a rather confounding paradox. Despite increasing prosperity, people in the West and developed societies as a whole are collectively facing an underlying existential crisis that seems to become more and more prevalent with each generation. Incredulously, most people seem to avoid talking about (or even recognizing) this perilous phenomenon, as if admitting its existence would somehow contribute to its grip on humanity.

Instead, the problem is frequently masked by an unrelenting pursuit of hedonism (that is, pleasure-seeking) that comes in a multitude of forms, whether it be through the heavy use of drugs, alcohol/partying, video games, pornography, fast food, entertainment, or even broader internet and social media use. These dopamine-inducing activities are becoming more and more common and, by virtue of our free market system (which exponentially encourages and rewards whatever produces the most money), are often used as a distraction and coping mechanism to avoid contending with the realities of life, if even subconsciously.

Admittedly, our increased prosperity has indeed led to a more complex and stressful life in many regards. The fact of the matter is that the more we have, the more we have to take care of. The more people there are, the more complex our political and governmental systems become and the more competition there is in all spheres of life. The faster our world operates, the faster we have to move to keep up with it. The more we learn as a species, the more our children are accountable for knowing and therefore are responsible for learning in school. Our undeniably impressive yet rather slow psychological evolution is not nearly fast enough to keep up with the rate at which the world is evolving.

There is no doubt that these factors of extreme stress and overload all contribute toward our perceived need to engage in extreme pleasure-seeking activities as a form of escape and relief. The ironic thing, however, is that these excessively pleasurable activities end up contributing toward a lessened ability to *deal* with the entailments of life to begin with. These activities often lead to an endless cycle that leaves us unfulfilled, apathetic, and, if not abandoning our responsibilities entirely, doing the absolute bare minimum to get by.

It is no wonder, then, that we have a mental health crisis on our hands. Accounting for the emergence of medications such as anti-depressants, increasing rates of depression, anxiety, and suicide (especially among millennials – broadly speaking, those born between 1985 and 2005) are indicative of an inability and/or unwillingness to deal with the entailments of modern life. Often, this is through no fault of their own. Underneath all of this, however, I believe that there is a more essential problem at the heart of this issue that serves as both a cause and a consequence of our pleasure-seeking mindsets: *a crisis of meaning*.

This notion is supported by the relevant psychological research, which cites that the increase in mental health issues in the United States can be attributed to "…cultural shifts toward extrinsic goals, such as materialism and status and away from intrinsic goals, such as community, meaning in life, and affiliation."[2] As is often the case, trends in the United States tend to reflect trends that occur elsewhere in the world, and other psychological literature confirms this mental health trend (and the reasons therefor) to also be the case in most of the Western world.[3]

If you were to ask the average person in Western society a question regarding why they do what they do, you'd be surprised at how shallow (if not wholly non-existent) their reasoning often is.

"Why are you in college/university right now?"
"Well, my parents want me to get a degree…"

"Why do you want to be a doctor?"
"Well, they make a lot of money and I want to be able to buy a nice car when I'm older."

"Why do you go to the gym every so often?"

"Well, I want to get a six-pack so I can look good on the beach and hopefully attract some girls."

"Why do you go to work every day?"
"Well, I need money to buy food and survive, quite frankly."

Then, you throw a hardball:

"Why do you live?"

Inevitably, you will see a noticeable display of hesitation. If they are brutally honest, they might say something like "I don't really know, to be honest." Alternatively, you might get something like "To have fun" or "To be happy." Most often, however, you will get a generic response that is rather insincere but is what they know would qualify as a socially acceptable or otherwise expected answer: "To help others, of course."

Looking at Western society today, it is quite evident that as a collective, we have lost true meaning and purpose, which I would argue is absolutely necessary in order to live a truly happy, fulfilling, and healthy life. Deep down, we all know this to be true, yet still have an immensely difficult time with establishing meaning in our own lives. This is not without good reason, though; finding meaning can be extremely difficult, which is precisely why philosophers who were likely much smarter than you or I have struggled with the problem for millennia.

It seems that in light of the way our current society operates we have largely foregone the search for meaning, whether through never considering it in the first place or searching for it and failing. This has left us with a dangerous collective existential foundation in nihilism; the belief, held consciously or unconsciously, that nothing truly matters in the grand scheme of things. Our civilization is grounded upon an astonishing contradiction; hoping and wishing that a collective belief in nihilism isn't the case, yet acting as if it is.

Chances are if you have picked up this book and read this far you yourself are either searching for meaning, have doubts about your own conception of meaning, and/or wish to enhance the sense of meaning you have already established for yourself. Pursuing meaning is perhaps among the most honorable pursuits in all of humankind and you are to be commended for doing so in an age when it is so tempting to abandon the quest. In order to find and establish a solidified sense of meaning, it is first necessary to understand how we got to this period of widespread nihilism in the first place. Having this understanding will allow you to subsequently solve for yourself what society as a whole is struggling with.

For this, we will take an extraordinarily interesting and enlightening chapter-long journey through humanity's history in the search for meaning. This will help you to understand the long path that human meaning has travelled and how we have arrived at our current dilemma. It's important to note that while the historical phases of meaning that I describe do intersect with each other in terms of their overall timeline, they do represent distinct and observable periods in which the noted concept of meaning was the predominant source at the time.

1

A Brief History of Meaning

The First Traces of Meaning: Mythology

Upon the emergence of modern humans about 150,000 years ago, our species (*homo sapiens*) still had yet to evolve to the point of being able to mentally consolidate an abstract concept such as 'meaning' in any noteworthy way. However, this is not to say that we did not live without purpose; as with all life forms, *survival* was a basic instinct towards which almost all of our actions were oriented. It is interesting to note that for the 140,000 years that we lived in what are called 'hunter-gatherer' societies up until approximately 10,000 years ago, primitive forms of morality (as it is currently conceptualized) *did* exist since the value of individual survival necessarily extended to that of the group as well.[4]

Hunter-gatherer societies typically consisted of a group of 30-40 individuals, although this number could grow up to around 200 if several bands of humans joined together at the same time. Historians and anthropologists have found that these groups were actually quite egalitarian and communal in nature due to the fact that all of the members depended upon each other to fulfill different roles within the division of labor. The group's survival also depended upon the cooperation of all members in almost every aspect of life.[5]

Selfishness was quite an absent trait in these societies, primarily because the notion of owning private property was precluded by the fact that the bands would frequently relocate after exhausting all of the resources in a given area of land.[6] In other words, any property that was 'owned' would have to be left behind very shortly after it was acquired since it was not sustainable for an extended period of time.

Insofar as early hunter-gatherer societies go, the only conception of *meaning* that can be extracted is very primitive and is primarily found in the importance of individual and group survival. Evolutionarily speaking, survival is of course spurred on by a natural desire to avoid pain. Meaning and purpose were therefore fulfilled merely by doing the things necessary to ensure the survival of the individual and the group, including cross-generational human survival through the process of reproduction.

Although there *is* some limited evidence of hunter-gatherers formulating ideas of supernatural beings and gods prior to this, about 14,000 years ago is when we begin to see substantial evidence of progress with regard to their conceptions of meaning since this is when more complex spoken language began to emerge.[7] At this point hunter-gatherers began attempting to explain *natural* phenomena by formulating *supernatural* explanations such as spirits and gods.

American author Robert Wright categorizes these supernatural explanations as belonging to four main groups: elemental spirits (those that inhabit inanimate objects), organic spirits (those that inhabit living things), ancestral spirits (spirits that come from the deceased), and high gods (one or more supreme gods that is of utmost importance, usually due to the fact that it was the 'creator' god).[8]

Now, why is this important for our sense of meaning, you might ask? The answer is mainly that this is the first evidence that we have for members of our species establishing a noteworthy system of meaning and purpose in their lives. According to these spirits and gods that they believed occupied the natural world, certain human acts were seen as being ethical and others as unethical. This gave the late hunter-gatherers a purpose beyond survival;

namely, pleasing the spirits/gods that supposedly occupied the world around them and that also had a preference as to how humans acted.

A useful example of this would be hunter-gatherers believing that a god started a thunderstorm because it was angry, for instance. The hunter-gatherers might witness a scary event such as a thunderstorm, attribute that scary event to a god that controlled that natural phenomena, look at what they had done differently in the recent past, and finally reason that it was those actions which had caused the god to become angry. This represented an early form of human beings seeking out patterns and trends within nature and deducing causes for anomalous events. These types of ideas presented humans with guidelines as to how they should act and what they should strive towards, and would serve as the foundation for what would later become known as 'mythology'.

Mythology, broadly defined, refers to collected narratives (or myths) of a given culture that often: attempt to explain natural phenomena through their personification as spirits or gods, serve as exaggerated accounts of historical events, and/or represent attempts to explain cultural rituals. Mythology often has the effects of fostering a sense of belonging among members of the culture, offering practical wisdom, and providing behavioral and moral guidelines to the society at large.

Perhaps the most popularized form of mythology is Greek mythology, which socioculturally unified Ancient Greece through its narratives of polytheism. Polytheism refers to the perceived existence of multiple gods, such as Zeus, Apollo, and Dionysus in Greek mythology, among many others. Greek mythology also contained narratives of mortal heroes whose actions were to serve as inspiration for humankind to aspire to.

The widespread belief in these tales and gods led Ancient Greece to construct not only a strong sense of meaning, but also of purpose, which was founded in a common moral code. This moral code used the myths of mortal human heroes as a symbol of how one should strive to act and myths of the gods as interpretations of what the supernatural deities *wished* for humans to do. Meaning and purpose were thereby founded in appeasing the gods, as they were for almost all cultures that engaged in a common mythology.

The transition from meaning and purpose being attached solely to survival towards more complex moral codes based in mythology would take approximately 140,000 years. The predominance of mythology as the primary source of meaning for humans would last until shortly after the Common Era began in the year 1 A.D. However, it is worthy to note that a relatively brief yet significant interruption in this trend did occur beginning around the 6th century BCE with the birth of what is called 'philosophy'. Ironically enough, this shift in human thought would occur in the very place where mythology arguably had one of the strongest holds; in Ancient Greece.

Meaning, Re-evaluated: The Birth of Philosophy

Beginning most significantly around the 6th century BCE, a new method of exploring the nature of the world and finding human meaning began to take hold in several geographical areas across the world (including Ancient Greece, China, India, and the Middle East, among others). This method was termed "philosophy", which translates literally as the "love of wisdom" (from the Greek *philos* and *sophia*, respectively).

As opposed to the largely inductive, speculative, and lore-based explanations of natural phenomena given by mythology, philosophy instead sought to provide explanations of the world around us through the use of our intellectual faculties and capabilities that had evolved immensely since the dawn of mythology. These faculties include concepts such as logical questioning, systematic representation, critical discussion, and rational argument, among others.[9]

While mythology attempted to explain the natural world using primitive and primarily supernatural explanations, philosophy began to use methods more akin to the *scientific method* we know of today by using rational thought, the logical process of deduction, and empirical observations of the world around us. Natural philosophy, in fact, served as the foundation upon which the sciences and most other intellectual methods of inquiry grew and developed.

While the beginning of philosophy is most commonly attributed to the Ancient Greeks of the 6th century BC (who primarily focused on natural philosophy and were aptly called the Pre-Socratics, including those such as Thales and Pythagoras), it is widely accepted that no individual captured the true essence of philosophy more so than a man named Socrates who lived from 469-399 BCE.

Socrates lived in the city-state of Athens in Ancient Greece, and was reportedly told by an oracle that he was the wisest man in all of Athens. After having conversed with those who were perceived to be the wisest men in Athens according to its citizenry, Socrates eventually came to a rather startling conclusion. He openly claimed that he was the wisest man in Athens *merely because he was aware of his own ignorance*; that is, he felt that he was aware of how much there was that he truly did not know.[10]

At this point, Socrates went on what could be termed as an 'intellectual crusade' throughout the city-state to question the basic assumptions and principles of Athenian citizens. He did this by using demonstrably impeccable logic to bring their moral and philosophical foundations into question, and often causing them to falter entirely in the process. To do this, Socrates used what was later deemed the *Socratic Method*; a conversational and argumentative strategy of deduction in which he would ask a series of questions that, when answered and agreed upon, would ultimately result in a conclusion that was contrary to the assumptions held by the individual being questioned.[11]

In essence, through strategic questions posed by Socrates and his interlocutor's subsequent agreement to certain propositions, the individual in question would eventually disprove their very own beliefs. This was done through the use of deductive logic by Socrates. In other words, if he could get the other individual to agree to a series of premises that lead to a conclusion contrary to their beliefs, they would then realize that they must necessarily agree to that given conclusion.

Through this crusade, Socrates inspired a city-wide re-evaluation of beliefs, even when it came to those who were perceived to be the wisest. Naturally, the rulers of the Ancient Greece did not take too kindly to his methods nor their results. In their view, questioning the core beliefs of Athenian citizens was akin to questioning the core beliefs of the city-state itself. Since the Ancient Greek population as a whole was largely homogenous in its belief in the Greek mythological figures and gods, there was a shared culture that allowed for coherent and more or less unanimously accepted political and moral systems.

Through the collective belief in this mythological foundation of philosophical, political, and moral thought, the population of Athens had engaged in a collective sense of meaning and purpose that they could aspire towards as a unit. Socrates' creation of micro-level tears in this foundation (if only through inspiring self-doubt and rational thought at the level of individuals), caused a macro-level threat to the city-state to be perceived by the government.

Consequently, Socrates was brought to trial by the government of Athens with two charges: corrupting the youth of Athens, and not believing in the gods of the city.[12] While the former is up to interpretation depending on if one views critical thinking as a positive or negative thing, the latter is quite interesting given that Socrates *did* partake in believing in the Greek gods, but was merely perceived to have caused citizens to question some of the basic underlying assumptions surrounding their existence and fundamental nature. Eventually, Socrates was sentenced to death, but his ideas and inspiration lived on through his students. Socrates' most notable student was Plato, who subsequently taught Aristotle, who, in turn, served as a mentor to Alexander the Great.[13]

Despite mythology still having a strong hold on the human population for centuries following their influence, philosophers like these (and others across the world, such as Zoroaster, the Buddha, and Confucius) would collectively put a massive dent in the way we humans conceptualized the pursuit of meaning. Values such as critical thinking, skepticism, logic, and objectivity would prove to be immensely valuable when establishing true meaning in our lives, and have perhaps never been as prevalent as they are at present.

To get to where we are today, however, the ideas of these philosophers would first have to contend with a rather sudden, unprecedented, and hugely significant threat that dominated our conception of meaning for nearly two millennia: religion. Although this source of meaning is declining in many parts of the world with respect to its relevance in peoples' lives, it still holds immense and unparalleled influence today.

An Unforeseen Phenomenon: The Rapid Emergence of Abrahamic Religion

As an academic field of study, the history of religion typically explores back as far as 3200 BCE with the emergence of writing.[14] Interestingly enough, the Ancient Greek mythology described in previous sections is often described by scholars as Ancient Greek *religion*. Even though modern religion is greatly distinguishable from ancient religion and mythology, the two are often conflated, much to the detriment of our understanding of the history of human meaning. This is not to say that the two concepts are entirely dissimilar, but there are indeed distinguishable characteristics that can allow us to understand the sources of human meaning more clearly and map out exactly how the concept has evolved over time.

Earlier, we defined mythology as "...collected narratives (or myths) of a given culture that often attempt to explain natural phenomena through their personification as spirits/gods, serve as exaggerated accounts of historical events, and/or attempts to explain cultural rituals." Religion, on the other hand, can be defined as "...a cultural system of designated behaviors and practices, worldviews, texts, sanctified places, prophecies, ethics, and/or organizations, that often relates humanity to supernatural, transcendental, and/or spiritual elements."[15] A helpful way to highlight the difference between the two, then, is that religion can have (and often *does* have) mythology implanted *within* it, but mythology often only serves as a *part* of a broader and more comprehensive religious system.

Early mythology, then, sometimes did have some *effects* of religion, whereby its adherents were familiar with its respective mythology, used the actions of heroes and gods as an aspirational ideal which sometimes informed their behavior, and performed rituals as per the perceived will of the gods. However, mythology often had a relatively weak hold over the people who lived within its sphere of influence for several reasons.

Firstly, it was polytheistic in nature, which often lead to competing interpretations of the will of each of the gods and the perception of competing interests among the gods themselves. As such, the peoples' conceptions of rules and moral/ethical systems was vague and rather unsolidified. Furthermore, mythology was able to retain relevancy only in small geographical areas due to technological and transportational barriers that existed during the time that it was most prevalent. Finally, there was a lack of interest and/or perceived necessity on behalf of its adherents regarding its spread to other societies.

Modern religion, however, is substantially greater in magnitude, scale, and comprehensiveness. It is not restricted to a small geographical area as mythology almost always was and it is significantly more systematic in nature. This systematic nature was made possible both through its monotheistic tendencies (which entail the belief in one singular and indisputable creator who sets the rules in each religion) and through the encouragement among its adherents for the spread of its ideas to people across the world.

Major religions almost always consist of a highly (and often politically) organized, widespread, and morally solidified belief system that is governed by a core holy book, which is often comprised of a complex collection of holy texts. It is these factors, in combination with its deeply philosophical nature and entailments that led has religion to constitute the single most impactful phenomenon and development with regard to the establishment of meaning in all of human history.

Following the rise of the early philosophers, it was unlikely that any new mythology would make exceptional headway in a reasonably large geographical area nor among a significant number of people. The natural philosophers had made an unprecedented amount of headway with regard to explaining natural phenomena. As a result, less and less of these phenomena were able to be used to infer the existence of some sort of god that was responsible for them since they had already been explained scientifically. This progressive and seemingly exponential phenomenon can be conceptualized as the *demystification of nature*.

In conjunction with the overwhelming power of critical thinking and logic, this process made the formulation of new mythologies increasingly difficult since they would henceforth be scrutinized and subject to careful scientific analysis and skepticism. Shortly following the emergence of philosophy, however, those who would begin to form the pillars of the three major monotheistic Abrahamic religions (Christianity, Judaism, and Islam) stumbled upon a brilliant concept. This came in the form of ensuring that their God is unfalsifiable and not subject to scientific scrutiny by placing it outside of nature and the realm of reality that we know. This way, there was no logical or empirical way to disprove its existence.

The three Abrahamic religions, as a collective, were named after Abraham, a key figure who played a very prominent yet differing role in each of the three religions. All three religions emerged at different times, yet they are all considered to be founded upon a belief in the same God (the God of Abraham), merely with different approaches with regard to His will and the historical interpretations of events.[16] Judaism is the oldest of the three religions, with its history going back as far as the second millennium BCE (in approximately 1500 BCE, although when accounting for the detrimental effect of conquests, its true growth is largely believed to have begun around 300 BCE).[17] Christianity began later in approximately 100 CE, while Islam had its start in approximately 600 CE.

Scholars consider Judaism, Christianity, and Islam to be the three 'Western' religions, insofar as the philosophical scholarly version of the term denotes 'having originated in a geographical area that is located west of the Indus River'.[18] It is worthy to note that the conventional conception of the term 'Western' will instead be used throughout most of this book (which broadly refers to the Americas and Europe; the areas of the world that are predominantly founded in Judeo-Christian philosophic traditions). Of course, other Eastern religions such as Buddhism and Hinduism were also prevalent at this time, but our primary focus is the Western world since it is where the crisis of meaning is most evident.

For our purposes, listing the fundamental tenets of each religion is not necessary, as most philosophically-engaged individuals have a basic understanding of what each religion entails. What *is* important, however, is understanding the importance of these three religions in establishing a sense of meaning and shifting humanity from deriving meaning in survival, mythology, or philosophical study. Major religions like these three (and most especially Christianity and Islam), spread rapidly and systematically, creating unparalleled influence on the philosophical foundations of millions (and eventually, billions) of individuals worldwide. This ushered in an age of religion serving as the primary source of humanity's perception of meaning.

Meaning in the age of these major religions was attached to a singular God. However, his will and evolution were interpreted differently in each religion's respective holy texts, which were widely accepted as being the official source of philosophical foundation/teachings, morality, ethics, and the historical events that shaped their doctrines. In all three religions, these holy texts were provided by God and his prophets/disciples, meaning that they served as revealed truths by a supernatural omnipotent, omniscient, and omnipresent creator who exists separate from this universe that He created.

Notably, God is portrayed as having the ability to intervene in worldly affairs in all three Abrahamic religions. Meaning is therefore to be found in acting in accordance with the expressed wishes of this creator who has endowed humanity with the gift of life, as listed in the respective holy texts. These texts outline precisely how humans were created and what living a good and moral life consists of. Therefore, meaning is to be found in having been created by a supernatural power and purpose is found in attempting to align oneself most closely with the guidelines listen in the holy texts (and thereby adhering to that creator's wishes).

The effect of this transition of human meaning has been profound. As political systems throughout the Western world evolved, religion served as a primary motivator for the expansion of empires and the conquest of territory. Imposing God's will and spreading his message to others also became key goals for each religion's adherents. The moral systems of empires were often grounded in the respective religions and as empires fragmented into nation-states, the leaders of these states conformed to religious doctrine and used them to inspire the laws that governed their territory. Judeo-Christian ideals largely inspired the foundation of North American, Central American, South American, and European philosophy, politics, and law, while Islam did the same for the Middle East and North Africa.

These notions are supported by the vast religious populations of these respective geographical areas. As of 2010, population research shows that Christianity is the religion of 77.4% of North American population, 75.2% of the European population, and 90% of the population of Latin America & the Caribbean.[19] Islam, on the other hand, accounts for a combined 93% of the Middle Eastern and North African population.[20]

This idea is further demonstrated through observing the religious population of the world as a whole. According to 2015 Pew Research, over 2.3 billion individuals worldwide identify as being Christian (31.2% of the world population), over 1.8 billion people identify as being Muslim (24.1%), and over 14 million individuals identify with Judaism (0.20%).[21] This means that in total, approximately 56% of the Earth's entire human population currently follows one of the three monotheistic Abrahamic religions at the time of writing.

This means that well over half of the entire world population likely derives its core sense of meaning from the perceived existence of one God and the holy texts that are derived from and/or inspired by Him. It is important to note that as per the listed methodologies of these studies, most were conducted using surveys in which people self-identified with one of the three religions, and therefore they do not take into account those who were merely *influenced* by them but do not overtly *self-identify* with one.

Never before in history has a singular source of meaning been so ubiquitous and homogenous among the human population than the rise of Abrahamic religion. Of course, while this collective source of meaning has inspired innumerable wars and conflicts due to its various interpretations, it has also inspired unparalleled societal and technological progress for the human species. Ironically enough, it is this exact progress that would eventually threaten the very legitimacy of these foundations of meaning.

The Renaissance and the Enlightenment

During the harrowing period of the Middle Ages which broadly spanned from approximately 400 CE to 1500 CE, humanity's dominant senses of meaning became quite oppositional in nature. The Middle Ages saw brutal religious conflicts and violent occupations, especially in the form of the Crusades and the responses to them (by Christians and Muslims respectively). Religious intolerance was rampant, and expressed itself in the form of the violent suppression of any alternative religious views, whether it was paganism/polytheism, perceived heresy, and/or opposing monotheistic ideas.

Human meaning and purpose in the more 'developed' world (mainly Europe and the Middle East) during the Middle Ages was principally derived from fighting for the religious views of one's respective empire, suppressing others for the sake of spreading religious doctrine, and conquering land for one's own idea of God. Notably, since the printing press was not invented until the mid-1400s and therefore the holy books could not be widely distributed to the masses, the interpretation of God's will was often left to the leader(s) of a given Empire's church or religious authority to decide and subsequently order their people to act upon instead of individuals being able to establish their own interpretation of the text.

Toward the end of these dark ages, from approximately from 1300 CE to 1700 CE, a new movement began in Europe which was eventually named the 'Renaissance' (literally translated from French as the *rebirth*). The Renaissance is largely considered to have served as an intellectual and cultural revolution of sorts. The revelations brought forth by the Renaissance sparked a societal reinvigoration of various creative elements of life including literature, philosophy, art, music, politics, science, and religion.

Following the devastating consequences of the religious wars of the Middle Ages and the peak of the Black Plague (which collectively killed between 100-200 million people during a time period in which the total world population likely never exceeded 500 million at any given point)[22/23], those remaining in Europe faced a period of relative wealth. This period of prosperity afforded them with the opportunity to reflect upon what exactly had gone so wrong in the centuries prior. This allowed for the investment of time and resources into intellectual and cultural pursuits, as well as the beginning of a widespread reorganization of political systems in an attempt to avoid the mistakes of the past.

In addition to major events such as the discovery of the New World (what is now North America) and the Protestant Reformation, a shift in focus led toward a return to the ideas of Ancient Greek and Roman philosophers, causing an intellectual 'rebirth' of society. The ideas of great thinkers of this period such as Leonardo da Vinci, Galileo Galilei, Nicolaus Copernicus, William Shakespeare, Petrarch, and Michelangelo, among many others, would cause the European population to re-evaluate its ideas about the meaning of life.

The renewed focus on scientific, artistic, philosophic, and humanistic pursuit during the Renaissance (which was most often still conducted under the inspiration of Christianity) would lead to a new period of intellectual growth that was unprecedented in human history and had effects that are still becoming ever more prevalent in today's world. Starting approximately after the year 1700, the 'Age of Enlightenment' began, sending cultural shockwaves across the human population. The developments of the Enlightenment caused a widespread re-evaluation of our conceptions of meaning, the effect of which was perhaps only matched in scale by the introduction of monotheistic religion.

The Enlightenment's principle impact is best encapsulated by looking at the ideas presented in the French philosopher Rene Descartes' work titled *Meditations on First Philosophy*. In this work, Descartes puts himself through an intellectual exercise in which he strips himself of all the preconceptions and beliefs that he has that he deems to be not grounded in *absolute* objective certainty, and attempts to build his knowledge back up by using only objective and indisputable truths. Throughout his initial meditations, Descartes realizes how much of his worldview was based in pure assumption that had never truly been properly evaluated, causing him to experience somewhat of an existential crisis when he realizes how little there is upon which he can begin to build his philosophical and intellectual foundations.[24]

This concept quite accurately symbolizes the experience of humanity upon the emergence of the foremost Enlightenment thinkers. Under the influence and inspiration of the early philosophers that were previously discussed (and whose ideas had been dwarfed by rise of monotheistic religion), humanity began a massive shift towards viewing objectivity, reason, and skepticism as foremost values in this new intellectual age.

Consequently, ideas and assumptions that had formerly been posited as truths were re-evaluated and challenged by some of the greatest thinkers of all time, including (but certainly not limited to) John Locke, David Hume, Immanuel Kant, Montesquieu, Jean-Jacques Rousseau, Voltaire, and Adam Smith. Humanity subsequently endured what can be described as a collective existential crisis and a widespread reorientation of values in light of new discoveries and worldviews based in objectivity.

The Enlightenment was therefore responsible for instilling new values and ideals in society such as liberty, progress, religious tolerance, constitutional government, and the separation of church and state. Following the Thirty Years' War from 1618-1648 (which began as a series of conflicts between Protestant and Catholic states and evolved into a larger European war among the great powers), the Peace of Westphalia was instated. This treaty formally established and recognized the inviolable sovereignty of nations for the first time in human history.[25]

This treaty would have the effect of reconstructing the political organization of Europe, which would later inspire the rest of the world's reorganization. This allowed each nation-state to form its own values and political organization, and made the Enlightenment values of constitutional government and the separation of church and state possible. Both during and as a consequence of the Enlightenment, numerous monarchies and states under religious/divine rule would eventually be overthrown and replaced with more secular regimes across Europe and the Americas. As we shall see shortly, this, in combination with the preeminent Enlightenment values of objectivity and reason, would have profound effects upon human meaning.

2

How We Arrived at the Crisis of Meaning

Our current crisis of meaning can be traced back to several distinct factors that were made possible by the historical progression that has been outlined so far. Insofar as I am able to discern, our crisis of meaning can mainly be attributed to five major trends that have taken hold since the Enlightenment. Notably, this is not to say that these five trends are inherently bad things in themselves, but merely to say that they *have* affected our sense of meaning in a significant way that we have hitherto been unable to meaningfully account for. The five major trends are as follows:

(1) The Fragmentation of Our Global System
(2) Widespread Immigration
(3) Our Increased Knowledge & Understanding
(4) Decline of Religious Thought & the Rise of
      Non-Religion
(5) Capitalism & Globalization

I – The Fragmentation of Our Global System

As aforementioned, the Peace of Westphalia combined with Enlightenment ideals such as secularism, religious tolerance, and the separation of church and state resulted in a massive rearranging of borders across the world, the effects of which are still evident today. This process included the fragmenting of previously massive empires and the overthrow of many absolute monarchies that were highly influenced (if not overseen by) the predominant church and theocratic governments that existed throughout the Western world.

These revolutionary changes perhaps most significantly began with the French Revolution in 1789. Religious regimes across the world were eventually replaced with republics and liberal democracies, which tended to embody not only the Enlightenment value of the separation of church and state, but often entailed the establishment of a written constitution that recognizes freedom of religion.

In effect, this process constitutionalized the value of religious tolerance and openness in numerous countries, even if they were considered to be distant end goals.

As a general rule in countries that are transitioning towards becoming more secular, constitutions (whether written or unwritten) have the effect of supplanting religious texts and holy books as the foremost authority when it comes to state organization, operations, and functions. They also enumerate and protect the highest values of the population as a whole. This essentially means that constitutions synthesize the will of the state's population into broader and more generic values that can apply to all individuals despite the immense variation and diversity of opinion with regard to meaning that is especially prevalent in diverse Western countries.

These countries and their populations therefore operate merely on *political* and *systematic* values that allow for a wide-range of interpretation as opposed to being based in deeper meaning and a foundational philosophy, despite many of the laws themselves being loosely grounded in Judeo-Christian ideals. This means that among the population there is no uniform consensus as to what the core meaning of life is; we as individuals are merely sharing the same land, resources, and political system by virtue of occupying the same geographical area. Collective meaning, then, exists only insofar as our actions serve the country in which we live, whether that be through economic contribution, adherence to the laws which we have collectively decided upon, or other functional methods. As such, philosophical consensus and unanimity is simply not to be found in these types of countries.

This problem is compounded by the fact that as geographical entities, nation-states are much smaller than what had typically existed in the past (principally expansive empires and the like). This naturally means that there are more territorial/political units worldwide, all of which now exercise their own sovereignty. As such, each state can establish its *own* value system that is representative of its population (based on demographic factors such as ethnicity, religion, affluence, etc.)

This state of affairs has the effect of rendering any sense of *universal* human meaning on a philosophical level as being nearly impossible to establish. Instead, each self-contained unit of (usually) millions of people instead establishes its own value system based on mere political and systematic utility. In these kinds of states, meaning naturally becomes viewed as an increasingly relativistic and abstract concept that has little to no official and/or overt government recognition.

This certainly serves as quite a stark contrast this to most modern nation-states in the Middle East and historical empires wherein the population is religiously homogenous (aside from differing denominational beliefs within the same religion, perhaps) and in which religion plays a crucial role in the political processes of the state. The collective meaning of these populations is instead grounded in unfalsifiable, nearly unanimously agreed upon, and cohesive metaphysical beliefs that form the basis of the state's culture, collective goals, and moral/ethical system. This comprises one of the major reasons why the West is experiencing such a substantial existential crisis even through a period of unmatched prosperity, while senses of meaning among people in the Middle East are largely unscathed and are even *flourishing* despite catastrophic humanitarian crises, immense conflict, and comparative scarcity on the whole.

II – Widespread Immigration

The benefits of immigration to both the immigrant and the country that hosts them are plentiful. Immigration often affords the immigrant with better living conditions and more life opportunities. It can also increase the productivity of the country, thereby raising the country's GDP and filling in shortages in specialized workforce areas. Younger immigrants can also help care for aging populations when there is a shortage of young people locally, which is especially the case in the Western world due to the Baby Boom following the Second World War.

Furthermore, in cases of significant immigration influxes, the host country is usually enriched by new altruistic values of cultural diversity, tolerance, more comprehensive human rights legislation, and innovation, among other things. Western countries are particularly open and popular destinations for immigration, and this is most especially the case in countries like Canada and the United States (which are referred to as a 'cultural mosaic' and a 'melting pot' with respect to each of their populations and immigration policies), but is increasingly becoming the case in European countries as well.

There is no doubt that the rising rates of immigration has certainly challenged our greater sense of meaning in several ways, however. As a given country's immigrant population increases, that country must necessarily make a certain extent of concessions to that population. These concessions often come in the form of increasingly secular governance, further religious tolerance, extended rights for that population (thereby conferring responsibilities upon the host country), and ensuring that the migrant/minority populations' influence remains relatively proportionate with their sizes relative to the rest of the country's population.

Essentially, this means that while a country may have once shared a collective sense of meaning founded upon a given religion's moral and philosophical tenets, the ability to retain that sense of meaning usually decreases as immigration increases. These religious tenets cannot be imposed upon the new religious minority population(s) that is comprised of immigrants, and are often challenged by new ones that are brought along with them. As a result, values become less and less grounded in core philosophy and instead become more predicated upon things like political utility, maintaining peace and good relations among the host and immigrant populations, and fulfilling the proper functionality of the state.

In a diverse Western country, all values and philosophical beliefs (provided they are deemed as being 'reasonable') hold equal status no matter if they are conflicting or not. Where there might have once been a unified sense of meaning in purpose among a country's population, there are now several differing and often *competing* interpretations of meaning that have equal status and legitimacy under the law. Younger generations that grow up in this kind of society are exposed to these numerous conceptions of meaning, which can make it difficult for them to solidify their own sense of meaning in a sea of differing and often equally plausible belief systems.

New ideas and ways of life brought over by the immigrant population also serve as intellectual and philosophical challenges to the dominant meaning-related narratives that a given society/country was founded upon.

Just as immigration has the effect of altering the composition of a formerly ethnically homogenous population, it also dilutes previously philosophically homogenous and coherent senses of meaning.

III – Our Increased Knowledge & Understanding

Perhaps the most impactful of trends towards our crisis of meaning as a species has been our rapidly increasing knowledge and enhanced intellectual capabilities. The intellectual journey that characterized Ancient Greece following the dawn of philosophy was renewed with the Enlightenment, and the discoveries that were made changed not only our efficiency and capabilities as a civilization, but also our worldview. Just as the findings of natural philosophy ate away at the foundations of mythology, the Scientific Revolution began to eat away at the foundations of meaning that we had once found in the monotheistic religions and has continued to do so exponentially ever since.

A noteworthy example of this knowledge-based phenomenon can be found in Nicolaus Copernicus' 1543 work titled *On the Revolutions of the Heavenly Spheres*, which proposed a heliocentric model of the solar system (that is, a solar system in which the Sun is the center and the planets orbit around it), which challenged the then-dominant narrative of geocentrism (in which the Earth was hypothesized to be located at the center of the solar system).[26]

Galileo Galilei's improvements to the telescope were later used by to support this idea in the early 1600s, causing him to be persecuted by the Roman Inquisition, found guilty of heresy, and sentenced to a lifetime house arrest. Heliocentrism was perceived by the court to be "foolish and absurd in philosophy, and formally heretical since it explicitly contradicts in many places the sense of Holy Scripture…"[27] despite, of course, being the scientifically accurate model of the solar system. The religious view that Earth and humans are the center of the universe and the most important of creations was severely jeopardized by these findings, and evidently served as a threat not only to our belief system but also to those who sought to defend it at all costs.

Of course, since then, a rapidly increasing number of other astronomical discoveries have called the religious worldview into question. The fact that there are *hundreds of billions* of galaxies, most of which consist of more than *one hundred billion* stars and *billions* of other planets (of which the Sun and Earth form but a mere pair) inevitably leaves us with a furthered astronomical worldview of relative insignificance. [28]

This is coupled with the fact that we have learned that the universe is relatively loosely ordered save for a few relatively consistent natural laws that are sometimes broken; it is quite chaotic, in fact. Planets including our own are frequently pelted (if not entirely destroyed) by asteroids, black holes inevitably swallow up surrounding planets and stars, galaxies frequently collide with one another due to gravity (including our own, which is set to collide with the Andromeda galaxy in the distant future)[29], and the likely theory about the universe's fate is that it will suffer an inevitable heat death in which all thermodynamic energy has been expended.[30]

Closer to home, our own star, the Sun, is fated to continue growing to the point where it swallows the Earth before dying and exploding into a supernova, long before which all life on Earth will have been burnt to a crisp (if it does not end due to another cause beforehand, of course).[31] These facts, among numerous others, call into question any notion of intelligent design of the universe and also have grave implications when it comes to finding meaning when such a grim fate awaits most, if not all, celestial bodies and life forms.

We also now know that while the universe began approximately 13.8 billion years ago, the Earth itself was formed about 4.5 billion years ago.[32] This serves as quite a contrast to most monotheistic stories that portray the formation of the universe and Earth as having been relatively instant and the age of the Earth itself merely being a few thousand years old.

In addition, the advancement of our knowledge about life itself has also not helped the case for meaning. We now understand that life began on our planet approximately 4 billion years ago, and that over 99% of all species that were ever 'purposefully created' have now perished and gone extinct.[33] Add to this Charles Darwin's discovery of the process of evolution and we see a much different story as to our origins. Through chaotic and entropic circumstances combined with the natural law of the survival of the fittest, the human species has emerged. It appears to be quite evident that we were, at the very least, not purposefully and instantaneously created as we currently are. Science has demonstrated that our origins and development occurred under a much different set of circumstances than those presented in the book of Genesis, for instance.

Coupled with these scientific advancements that have helped us to better understand the world and the natural processes around us, philosophic ideas have also created immense challenges for establishing a sense of meaning. While we previously used religion as a collective foundation for meaning as a species, powerful philosophical ideas have shaken this foundation from beneath us. To postulate one of the many thousands of challenging ideas and theories that we have developed over the centuries, let us examine the *Problem of Evil*. In its logical formulation, it operates as follows:

1. God exists.
2. According to the doctrines of all three Abrahamic religions, God is perceived as being omnipotent (all-powerful), omnibenevolent (perfectly moral) and omniscient (all-knowing).
3. An omnipotent being has the power to prevent evil from coming into existence.
4. An omnibenevolent being would want to prevent all evils.
5. An omniscient being knows every way in which evils can come into existence, and knows every way in which those evils could be prevented.
6. A being who knows every way in which an evil can come into existence, who is able to prevent that evil from coming into existence, and who wants to do so, would prevent the existence of that evil.
7. If there exists an omnipotent, omnibenevolent and omniscient God, then no evil exists.
8. However, evil exists.[34]

Since this formulation is logically sound, it necessarily leads to one of four troubling conclusions:

1. God is not omnipotent.
2. God is not omnibenevolent.
3. God is not omniscient.
4. God does not exist.

It is numerous philosophic and logically troubling philosophical ideas like these that, in addition to the accelerated advancement of our scientific knowledge, have thrown a wrench into humanity's traditional and longstanding foundations of meaning that have historically been grounded in religious thought.

Our rapidly increasing knowledge in the realm of technology has also further compounded these effects. Not only has technology enabled us to make the aforementioned discoveries, but it has also created new methods of communication so that these ideas can be spread at a comparatively rapid rate. Prior to the invention of the printing press in the mid-1400s, it was extraordinarily difficult to share challenging ideas much further than a local community due to technological limitations that were coupled with the frequent acts of suppression by religious authorities.

With the emergence of the printing press, books containing these ideas could be written and distributed to a fairly larger geographical area with fewer limitations. Now, however, the internet serves as an unparalleled mechanism through which challenging ideas and knowledge can be spread and ubiquitously known across the world without much capability for interruption or restrictions. Consequently, it has become increasingly difficult for a given society or culture to remain immune to status quo-shattering ideas, knowledge, and shared understandings.

IV – The Decline of Religious Thought & the Rise of Non-Religion

This fourth trend - the rise of secularism, non-religion, atheism, and agnosticism - serves both as a consequence and a compounding agent to our increased knowledge as a species. Atheism and agnosticism have rapidly grown as plausible worldviews, and, given the aforementioned factors regarding our increased knowledge, it makes sense why this has happened. In fact, Pew research shows that education is negatively correlated with religious views on the national level. In other words, the more educated a country's population is, the less religious it tends to be (granted, economic factors do also contribute to this trend).[35]

The more that we learn, the more that many of the entailments of the Abrahamic religions appear to be increasingly unlikely and the less substantiated their presented conception(s) of meaning appear to be. We have increasingly becoming more capable of instead explaining the natural world around us using the scientific method and secular study. As such, the need to appeal to previously dominant religious ideas for epistemological guidance appears to be rapidly diminishing.

A 2002 study demonstrates the validity of this notion through analyzing shifts in religious attitudes among the world population over a period of just over a century (from 1900-2002). In terms of the number of people that self-identify as having one of the two philosophical worldviews, non-religion and atheism have proportionally made immense gains relative to Christianity and Islam, the world's two largest religions. Using rounded numbers, the Christian population of the world in 1900 was approximately 558 million, which grew to 2.05 billion in 2002 (a growth rate of 367%). The Muslim population of the world in 1900 was 200 million, which grew to 1.24 billion in 2002 (a growth rate of 620%). The non-religious population in 1900 was 3 million, which grew to 781 million in 2002 (a growth rate of 25,812%). The atheist population in 1900 was 226,000, which grew to 151 million in 2002 (a growth rate of 66,727%).[36]

As of 2012, the worldwide combined secular, nonreligious, atheist, and agnostic population is at approximately 1.2 billion, which accounts for 16% of the total world population (as opposed to the 0.2% of the world population that it comprised in the year 1900).[37] As per Pew Research, this collective nonreligious population is expected to decline slightly to about 13% of the world's population by 2050. This projected decline is largely attributed to this demographic's extremely low birth rates (about 1.7 children per woman) relative to religious demographics (such as the 3.1 children per woman birth rate of Muslims).[38]

Quite ironically and despite this projected *worldwide* decline, nonreligious populations are expected to *increase* in proportion in both North America and Europe by 2050. This serves as evidence that the once collective sense of meaning found in Christianity across the Western world has faltered, while that of the Middle East founded in Islam, for instance, has remained relatively stable. According to the Pew Forum on Religion and Public Life, by 2050 the nonreligious population in North America is expected to account for 27% of North America total population (up from 17.1% as in 2010), and 23% of Europe's total population (up from 18% as in 2010).[39]

Interestingly enough, this research also shows that in the United States, each successive generation of the population has consistently become less and less religious. As a simple example, 8% of those born before 1928 identified as being religiously unaffiliated in 2014, compared to 35% of those born between 1981 and 1996. This trend also appears to be prevalent across most of the Western world. [40]

Although religious populations are growing in a strictly numerical sense, it is important to reflect upon the populations' subjective sense of religious identity as well, since this can give us a better idea of exactly how attached an individual is to their own foundational sense of meaning. While the Muslim world as a whole appears to have a rather consolidated sense of meaning and a strong sense of connection to the Islamic faith, the Christian-founded Western world is witnessing a massive decline in the subjective relevance of Christianity and religion as a whole in peoples' lives.

Pew research conducted from 2008-2017 shows that the average percentage of people (averaged by country) who believe religion to be *very important* to their lives across Europe is 23%, and across North America is 42%, which starkly contrasts with the 73% in the Middle East/North Africa and 89% in Sub-Saharan Africa. If you pair each of the two geographical areas and average these percentages, it results in 32.5% for North America/Europe and 81% for the Middle East/Africa, a cumulative difference of 48.5%.

What is incredibly significant is that while the percentage of people that find religion to be very important in their lives differs by 48.5% across the two groups of geographical areas, the difference between them with regard percentage of people who affiliate with a religion in general is only approximately 20%. This demonstrates that while people might identify as being Christian in the Western world, this often might reflect their upbringing or sense of group identification but is less reflective of their *actual* commitment or level of belief in Christianity. This notion is also reflected in hugely differing rates of prayer and church attendance across the two groupings.[41]

These population demographics and ideological shifts are also reflected in the widespread and increasing popular discourse in the West that surrounds and calls into question the validity, viability, and utility of religious thought. Notably, intellectual discourse is of course to be encouraged, since any major belief system should be closely examined and subject to scrutiny to avoid blind belief, which can be exceptionally dangerous. This broadly anti-religious intellectual revolution of sorts has both prompted and been inspired by the rise of those who are colloquially referred to as the "New Atheists".

The New Atheists are prominent public intellectuals such as Sam Harris, Richard Dawkins, the late Christopher Hitchens, and several others who publicly endorse and advocate for the end of religious thought and the embracing of atheism as a worldview. Individuals like these have had extraordinary influence through their public talks, debates, books, and multimedia appearances. They serve as representatives of this new cultural and philosophical shift in human meaning, and simultaneously help to foster the extent to which it thrives.

To give you an idea of the influence of these relatively new ideas apart from shifting religious demographics, it is also worthy to note just how widespread they have become. Sam Harris' 2004 book, *The End of Faith*, for instance, immediately entered the New York Times Best Seller list at number four upon its release and remained on the list for a total of 33 weeks. Christopher Hitchens' 2007 book *God is Not Great: How Religion Poisons Everything*, on the other hand, reached number two on the Amazon bestsellers list within a week and reached number one on the New York Times Best Seller list in three weeks. Perhaps most notably, Richard Dawkins' 2006 book *The God Delusion* has sold over 3.3 million English copies thus far and ranked number two on the Amazon bestsellers list (upon which it remained for 51 consecutive weeks).[42/43]

Where thinkers like these have perhaps had the most cultural and intellectual influence, however, has been on online media platforms such as the ever-growing Youtube video-sharing website. Listed below are the results from adding up just the total views of merely the top 25 most-viewed videos that appear when one searches the names of the three aforementioned public intellectuals (out of thousands upon thousands of results). Only the videos which contain ideas pertaining to the supremacy of atheism as an intellectual position over other alternatives are included in these results. Keep in mind that these are just three individuals who represent a small *fraction* of public atheist thinkers whose ideas have recently become widespread and heavily influential:

- Richard Dawkins: 70+ million views in top 25 (over 291 videos with over 100,000 views each)[44]
- Christopher Hitchens: 57+ million views in top 25 (over 303 videos with over 100,000 views each)[45]
- Sam Harris: 45+ million views in top 25 (over 234 videos with over 100,000 views each)[46]

Given that Youtube's most popular age demographic in the Western world is the 18-34 age group, it is likely that these ideas are also disproportionally reaching younger people.[47]

All of this is not to say that those in the nonreligious/atheist/agnostic camp *cannot* find a deep sense of meaning (as this is certainly not the case), nor is this to make a normative judgment with regard to this trend. However, this rise in a nonreligious demographic *does* serve as a challenge to the *status quo* with regard to finding human meaning, which has predominantly been located within the Abrahamic religions since their respective inceptions. For nearly two millennia, well over half of the human population has found meaning in these monotheistic religions, and the rapid rise of the worldwide nonreligious population primarily serves as a symptom (but also one of many causes) of a massive crisis of meaning, especially among the Western world where it is most prevalent.

V – Capitalism & Globalization

Although more primitive and locally-based forms of capitalism existed for centuries prior, modern global capitalism is largely accepted to have emerged in the early 20th century following the Industrial Revolution, and was spurred on by the exponential process of globalization. Capitalism, of course, is an economic system based on private ownership of the means of production and their operation for profit, as opposed to state/government ownership. Core features of capitalism include private property, wage labor, voluntary exchange, a price system, competitive markets, and free trade. The emergence of capitalism as a global economic system has had surprisingly profound effects upon human conceptions of meaning worldwide, and especially in the areas of the world in which it most flourishes most.[48]

For those who are wondering what in the world economics could possibly have to do with human meaning, consider the following: our economic system is what shapes how our society functions, including what jobs are available, the level of equality or inequality experienced, and the level of comfort with which one is able to live. Our own financial status is capable of, at least in part, determining our worldview. As a simple example, someone who is able to comfortably afford to feed themselves and their family is likely to have a more positive outlook on life than someone who is struggling in poverty and unable to provide for their family. This idea is substantiated by ample evidence conveying a positive correlation between the wealth of a given country and its citizens' happiness and sense of purpose.[49]

In a capitalist system, providers of goods and services are able to operate relatively freely with regard to what they sell, at what price they sell it, and to whom they sell. Instead of these factors being dictated or limited by the government, business owners are instead constricted by competition. If businesses do not have a competitive product or service at a competitive price, they are not going to be able to last against competitors and accrue a significant enough profit that allows the business to keep operating successfully. Furthermore, to state the obvious, if a business does not offer products/services that are valued by consumers, it will not be in business very long. As such, businesses first strive for the creation of a worthy product (also known as value creation), before then attempting to attract the attention of consumers (through the process of marketing).

Over time, then, the capitalist system gravitates towards creating better and better products at increasingly better prices since the competition fosters innovation in order to outdo competing businesses. Through this competitive process, capitalism has done wonders worldwide in terms of providing food and comfort to billions of people who might have otherwise not been able to survive and has also led to revolutionary technological advances.

However, this same economic process can also result in consumers who are overloaded with the biggest and best of things advertised to them at a dizzying rate. One can just look at any computer screen, television screen, or the downtown streets of any metropolitan area to see striking evidence of this phenomenon. In addition, there is a central problem with this process with regard to finding a sense of meaning - capitalist systems also foster distraction and hedonism, the likes of which have never been seen before.

The process of value creation, as the name suggests, seeks to create a product or service that consumers want. Unfortunately, at our core, humans tend to instinctively want things that, if unchecked by a deeper sense of meaning (upon which our values are based) and if provided through an unmoderated forum, can ultimately lead to harm. Obvious examples of this include, sex, pleasure, novelty, and food, among many others.

More than ever before, shallow materialistic values like these are able to be met instantaneously and to the most extreme degrees by products and services that are widely and easily available. These wants (that often develop into perceived needs) are also constantly bombarding our minds through unceasing advertisements, which slowly begins to erode our individual and collective sense of meaning in favor of meeting them as soon and as often as possible. This process has therefore established shallow values in the population that have transcended and overthrown previously dominant and more worthwhile senses of meaning.

Although there are many obvious examples of this (including fast food and status-enhancing purchases), I would like to take a deeper look at one that is perhaps less obvious and that I think adequately illustrates this problem: internet pornography. Internet porn is an exponentially growing and lucrative phenomenon, and for good reason. Sex is perhaps our most basic instinctual desire aside from things strictly necessary for survival such as oxygen, water, and food. Though the reasoning for this is likely more multifaceted and complex, at its core sex is the means to ensure our long-term survival as a species through propagation and reproduction and is therefore of prime importance in our biological evolution.

The concept of pornography has evolved from black and white pictures in the back of a purchasable magazine to high definition, high production, and instantly-accessible video content of an infinite and diverse supply on any device that is able to connect to the internet. This evolution has occurred within the short span of a few decades. The use of porn, then, has naturally grown exponentially and is now used weekly or more often by a strong majority of those aged 13-24, and especially by males.[50] The demand for porn is so strong that it has more or less precluded the possibility of any kind of major intervention to moderate its production or subsequent use.

The use of porn activates the reward centers of the brain and floods the brain with pleasure chemicals such as dopamine at levels that are absurdly high compared to what has previously been possible apart from the use of chemical drugs. Naturally, then, porn has become the center of a multitude of scientific studies many of which are founded in a very simple phenomenon.

Interestingly enough, studies with male rats have shown that repeated sexual encounters with the same female rat leads to the male rat becoming less and less excited over time. However, if a new female rat is introduced into the mix, the male rat's sexual performance and pleasure levels consistently ramp back up again (and this is of course repeatable with each novel female). This study is repeatable with numerous kinds of mammals, including humans, and the phenomenon is commonly referred to as the "Coolidge Effect". Since repeated things produce less and less of a reaction in our brains, porn immediately meets the need for novelty and sexual excitement that is evidently inherent in much of animal psychology at a *perceived* low cost.[51]

What does porn do to solve this natural numbing effect, exactly? The answer is simple: it allows people to 'engage' sexually with an endless number of new specifically selected people each and every day. Due to the nature of capitalism, the individuals featured in porn have increasingly become more and more sexually attractive (through unnatural selection in order to achieve better value creation on behalf of a given porn production company that is competing with others), often to the point of being unattainable without substantial cosmetic surgeries. Just as repeated encounters breeds a psychological longing for novelty, so too does the daily use of porn, along with further reinforcing and strengthening that longing.

Naturally, the level of addiction that this creates is unparalleled by anything with the lone exception of some hyper-addictive drugs. Numerous studies have also shown that regular users of porn increasingly delve into more and more shocking kinds of porn in order to get as strong of a reaction each time (and, as per the laws of the free market, these categories and genres are delivered to meet the demand).[52]

Quite frankly, the human brain is simply not wired for this level of stimulation. In the real world, sexual partners have historically been rare, sexual attractiveness is widely variant, and monogamous behaviour served as the standard for at least several centuries now. Understandably, much scientific research has shown that regular use of porn can contribute toward libido loss and poor sexual performance in situations that *don't* involve porn, in addition to depression, anxiety disorders, social anxiety, lack of confidence, adultery, marital/relationship issues, attention and working memory issues, sexually deviant behaviours, the objectification and mistreatment of women…the list goes on and on.[53] While feeling pleasure usually serves as reward from achieving something substantial, porn instead allows an individual to receive a usually 'unearned' dose of pleasure chemicals the likes of which is nearly unparalleled in any natural sense and rewards nothing but sitting on the couch and clicking a few buttons.

The rise of internet pornography serves as an excellent metaphor for what has happened in our capitalist system; the hypercompetitive value creation process has evolved to the point of advertising (and providing) extremities of every sort that are increasingly addictive and harmful. Fast food has become increasingly affordable and tasty, while healthy food remains expensive and is barely palatable to those who regularly eat the former. The news media is predicated on providing the most shocking headlines possible, leading to an oversaturation of negative and sensationalized news for the sole purpose of grabbing attention.

Similarly, across the internet you will see the most attractive people, the richest people, the most famous people, the most successful people, the most beautiful of places, the most excessive abundances of materialism, and the most impressive sports feats plastered everywhere. The internet is based on quick highlight reels and rapid-fire exciting moments. As a whole, everything in this system appears to be predicated upon successive dopamine hit, after dopamine hit, after dopamine hit.

We then might decide to temporarily return to a healthy, wholesome, and otherwise fulfilling lifestyle and somehow everything seems dull, unexciting, and uninspiring. Our attention spans are the lowest that they have ever been and are decreasing quickly. The only thing that excites and motivates us is to be found in events such as purchasing something, doing drugs, drinking alcohol, or scrolling through the internet's endless content that shows the extremities of every aspect of life. The extent of meaning for millions worldwide has merely become about pursuing hedonistic desires and distracting themselves from the realities that they are intended to face.

The ironic thing is that while hedonism is pursued so strongly in Western societies despite its severe consequences, it is arguable that in a sense it does not bring any substantive benefits to the individual pursuing it. Much research has been done into what is termed the 'hedonic treadmill', a psychological theory that posits that as a person receives non-meaningful positive results (such as making more money, for instance) expectations and desires rise in tandem, which results in no net or permanent gain in happiness.

As we know, this also applies to the pursuit of physical pleasure. As we take more drugs, for instance, our tolerance rises and we require more and more to reach the same levels of pleasure we felt previously. This process, then, is akin to walking on a treadmill; although you are putting in the effort, in reality you are moving nowhere. In fact, as you tire you have to continue to progressively put in more effort just to stay in the same place.

A prime example of this phenomenon is that of our celebrity culture. Celebrities represent the peak of hedonistic pursuit since they have everything that those who pursue shallow pleasures wish for. This is perhaps a significant reason why they are so revered in the first place. Celebrities have immense wealth, fame, power, and influence, among many other things; everything the average person could every want, materialistically speaking. Despite this, they have alarmingly high rates of mental health issues, breakdowns, and/or drug addictions, and there is no evidence that they are happier than the average person on the whole. Not only does this serve as a clear indicator of the veracity of the hedonic treadmill theory, but it also goes to show that there is clearly something that is missing in their lives despite apparently having everything that most people could ever hope to have.

What appears to be missing in most cases like these is a true sense of meaning and purpose. After all, if these two things are found and acted upon, people tend not to throw their lives down the drain. Instead, a majority of celebrities seem to revolve their lives around making wild purchases without necessarily having to worry about maintaining them or paying them off. It is likely that they eventually realize that in order to sustain the things that they have, they have to keep maintaining a public presence and doing things that they might realize are not meaningful to them. They are then left with a daunting choice: either keep doing something that fails to fulfill them, or lose all the materialistic things in which they have placed their happiness. Not even having everything that most people in

Western society strive for fulfills these types of individuals. In fact, statistically speaking, it seems to be a *detriment* to many of them. This apparent paradox constitutes something that is certainly worth thinking quite deeply about.

For many people across the Western world, it is not entirely their fault that they succumb to these pursuits. After all, they are constantly bombarded by the psychologically-rewiring hedonistic phenomena all around them from birth and are born into a society in which the glorification of those of the highest status who have climbed the hedonistic ladder is commonplace. The ultimate aspirations in today's Western world are things such as having the most money, the most attractive partner(s), and the nicest cars.

It is certainly not easy to escape from these desires, and no matter how often people are told about their consequences, they often refuse to give them serious thought or consideration. Admittedly, this is quite understandable. A psychological wiring that prioritizes these desires makes it very difficult to escape them, since most of them come very close to constituting addictions. This is combined with the fact that we are societally accustomed to them since the pursuit of these things is now the norm (if you have not had sex, drank alcohol, done drugs, and watched porn before the age of sixteen, you are considered an absolute *weirdo* by the standards of today's high school peers).

These factors are further coupled with the unwillingness to face how poorly one has lived through fear of guilt (or realizing how much has been lost), the effort that it takes to live with limited hedonism, and the constant pressure and temptation surrounding us nearly 24/7. It is no wonder why our world has been consumed by the art of physical and mental consumption.

Not only has meaning become increasingly harder to find, but we now live in a world that does its best to distract us from even considering it until we encounter a personal crisis from which our hedonistic desires and habits cannot save us (and we often know this to be the case). In these moments, we *know* what must be done and we have an intuition as to how life *should* be lived to resolve the problems that we are facing. However, a strong majority of us sink deeper into denial and hedonistic pursuits in an attempt to mask and distract us from our problems. Some of us, however, recognize, accept, and act upon the deeper problem before it is too late; *a lack of foundational meaning and purpose in our lives.*

3

Defining Meaning and Purpose in Your Own Life

With an understanding of both the history of human meaning and why the West as a whole is currently undergoing a crisis of meaning, it is now time to reflect upon and further develop your *own* sense of meaning. To begin, we will first examine what exactly the terms 'meaning' and 'purpose' mean to you, and what distinctions set them apart from one another. In order to find our own meaning and purpose, we of course have to know what exactly these terms mean to us as *individuals* so that we know what exactly it is we are searching for and/or feel that we are lacking in our lives. Establishing your own definitions for these two terms will allow you to exercise your free will and individual agency in determining what it is you live for and are trying to achieve in the future. While there are such things as collective senses of meaning and purpose that we have as a species, for many reasons understanding your own individual meaning and purpose is becoming increasingly important in the Western world.

As explained in the previous chapters, Western society as a whole is undergoing a crisis of meaning. There are many complicated factors that have contributed to this, but the end result is obvious and very apparent. Whereas the strong majority of us once shared a collective sense of deep philosophical meaning to which our governing bodies could aspire and lead our communities, the political fragmentation of our world and the interspersing of populations that hold different (and often competing) senses of meaning has caused us to default to mere *functional* values for the sake of achieving some semblance of organization despite conflicting worldviews.

Even during the age of mythology, when both meaning and the human population were arguably in their most fragmented states, communities existed so independently of one another that they could each adhere to their collective senses of meaning without interruption. Our increasingly globalized world has precluded the possibility of existing within this kind of communal bubble, however. In what seems to be an exponential process of the interspersing of populations and values, collective philosophical meaning has become all but lost.

Most of the laws and political systems of democratic societies (which comprise nearly all of the Western world) serve as temporary expressions of the collective functional values of the current population as a whole. These are, by the very nature of democracy, subject to frequent and rapid change and evolution. They are impermanent, largely shapeless, inconcrete, malleable, and are grounded in nothing short of political, legal, and sociocultural utility.

These expressions of value, when drafted into legislation and subsequently enforced, *do* help to keep society functioning at a basic level, but they do little to quell the ubiquitous human thirst for a deeper collective meaning and purpose that we have searched for as a species for millennia. As such, meaning is instead increasingly becoming a fundamentally individual pursuit. Establishing your *own* sense of meaning (while still operating within the political and legal confines of the system in which you live, of course) is integral in a world where your society or country as a whole is devoid of a coherent philosophical foundation.

Finding one's meaning and purpose is an exceptionally difficult task; after all, there is a reason our species has been in pursuit of them for so long. If we start with the basics and gradually build our sense of meaning up, however, you might be surprised as to how easy and deeply fulfilling this pursuit can be. So let us begin by first establishing definitions of 'meaning' and 'purpose' as they pertain to your own life. In order to define such abstract and important terms, it is incredibly useful to look at how meaning and purpose have traditionally been defined by human beings so that you can use these conceptualizations as a general guideline and a basis upon which to build your own understanding. After all, as Isaac Newton famously said: "If I have seen further it is by standing on the shoulders of Giants."[54]

Understanding the Concept of 'Meaning'

When accounting for the intended context which we are using to discuss it, the word 'meaning' is defined by the Merriam-Webster dictionary as "…a significant quality; especially: the implication of a hidden or special significance."[55] There is nothing quite like using the dictionary to help us find the meaning of life, am I right? On a more serious note, the meaning of life, according to this definition, would be "The most significant quality of life, which often holds hidden or special significance." Not a bad starting point, and surprisingly accurate if I do say so myself.

When we ask the question "What is the meaning of life?" we are asking a question that our species has asked since the inception of its capacity for reflective thought and that *no one* has ever answered with objective certainty nor with indisputable empirical evidence. Therefore, insofar as the meaning of life has not yet objectively been proven, is not overtly obvious by any means, and has been debated for millennia, it is indeed 'hidden'. The meaning of life can also easily be considered as being 'special', as life is certainly not a standard nor ordinary phenomenon given its apparent rarity. Finally, and perhaps most importantly, the meaning of life in some way grants *significance* to our existence. If our existence was not significant in some substantial way, then, naturally, it would be *insignificant*. If life was wholly insignificant, the existence of inevitable pain, suffering, and tragedy would necessarily make life not worth living in most cases.

Meaning, then, according to this definition, adds a sort of significance to life that makes it worth living despite the inevitable pain and suffering that we will endure. This corresponds directly with our historical search for meaning, since humans who have pursued an understanding of meaning in a significant way have often considered it to be something hidden, profound, and deeply philosophical in nature. Throughout history, the consensus has largely been that since a deep sense of meaning is not to be found through objective examination, it must in some sense be either be objective yet metaphysical (that is, beyond our current knowledge or understanding of the universe), or subjective (that is, relative to each individual's perception) in nature.

Looking at human life, we can indeed see traces of special significance all around us through objective observations that, while not necessarily indicative of an inherent meaning, do contribute towards our overall sense of significance. Looking at the sheer unlikelihood of our existence and its complexity is indeed a humbling and quite awe-inspiring exercise, for instance. Although it is wildly ambitious to put an actual number to it, many scientists have tried and have estimated the odds of life forming on Earth to about 1 in 10^{40} to 10^{400} (that is, the number "10" followed by forty to four-hundred zeroes).[56]

In addition to this, when looking at the unlikelihood of our existence as a life form you must also factor in the odds of a planet existing that is capable of sustaining life, and the conditions that must be present to allow this to happen. First, the planet must exist in the right location of a galaxy (not too far from the center, but not too close either) and in the right *type* of galaxy (one that is not too dense, nor has too much radiation, nor has an eccentric orbit). Second, the planet must orbit at the right distance from its star (in the small so-called "Goldilocks Zone" where liquid water can exist) and must orbit the right *type* of star (including relevant factors such as its size, metallicity, stability, and the fact that it cannot be a binary star – which approximately half of all stars are).[57]

The planet's solar system must also have the right number of planets and type of planets. This would include having small and rocky planets closer to the star, and bigger gaseous planets further from the star (to emit strong gravitational pulls that protect the smaller planets from asteroids, among other benefits). Finally, the planet has to have a continuously stable orbit, must be of the right size, and would ideally have plate tectonics and a large satellite moon.[58]

Out of the 3825 exoplanets (that is, planets that exist outside of our own solar system) that NASA has discovered thus far,[59] about 50 *potentially* fall within the mere requirements of being within their respective stars' goldilocks zone, having a rocky composition, and being of the right size.[60] In other words, these ~50 planets merely meet three of *numerous* other requirements, most of which are even less likely.

Finally, we must factor in that the process of biological evolution had to have occurred in the way that it did (again, something that is extraordinarily unlikely) to be able to get us to the point of intelligent life. Not only is the evolution of our species a truly wonderful, humbling, and seemingly mystical phenomenon that provides an instance sense of significance to any who study it, but it also tells the tale of the billions-of-years-long journey that life has endured and survived. In fact, just 75,000 years ago the human species is theorized to have almost went extinct around when a supervolcano in present-day Indonesia erupted and caused a population bottleneck to the point where there were less than 10,000 individuals alive on Earth.[61] Our continued existence, intellectual capabilities, and the fact that we are living in the most prosperous age in human history is, at the very least, immensely *statistically* significant.

Since our chemical composition is nearly identical to that of our galaxy and all matter is made up of elements that stars served as a factory to create, it is also apparent that we are very much part of the universe itself. As the late Carl Sagan once said, "The cosmos is within us. We are made of star-stuff. We are a way for the universe to know itself."[62] In other words, we are the medium through which the unimaginably massive and incredible universe gains self-awareness and understanding. This is a truly humbling thought, and it is precisely observations like these that allow us to truly see the special significance and meaning of our lives. Of course, these kinds of observations are made through the exercise of innate curiosity and knowledge-seeking, which allow us to acquire a sense of meaning and understanding of the inconceivable wonders that surround us.

Understanding the Concept of 'Purpose'

The interrelationship between meaning and purpose is indeed quite interesting. If you have a sense of meaning, you necessarily have a purpose. Likewise, if you have a true purpose, this necessitates the existence of a foundational sense of meaning. Due to this mutual dependence on their behalves, finding a definitional distinction between the two terms can be quite challenging indeed. The Oxford dictionary defines our contextual use of 'purpose' as follows: "The reason for which something is done or created or for which something exists" and/or "A person's sense of resolve or determination."[63]

Whereas 'meaning' seems to pertain more to a foundational *significance* with regard to life, 'purpose' seems to imply either a *reason* with regard to why life (or the universe) exists and/or a *reason* for living in a particular way. Put simply, meaning prompts the question "Why do I live?" while purpose prompts the question "In what way should I live and why should I live that way?" Notably, meaning is arguably more foundational in nature since you must first have a reason to live before then choosing to live in a particular way.

A conception of purpose that I find extraordinarily useful in my own life is inspired by ideas from the Greek philosopher Aristotle in his work titled *Nicomachean Ethics*. When considering the kinds of things that exist in the natural world, Aristotle classified them into a hierarchy of nature divided into four parts: *mineral, vegetative, animal,* and *human.* Aristotle argued that something's purpose ultimately depends on which category it belongs to.

According to Aristotle, Mineral things are those that are lifeless and inanimate. Without sentience, their purpose is to be utilized by those things which live. The Vegetative category refers to things such as plants and insects, with their purpose being to survive and for plants to fulfill their function of supplying oxygen which most other life forms also require to survive. An Animal's purpose is to survive, reproduce (through the basic function of seeking pleasure), and help other living beings survive, especially those of their own species. Notably, the Animal's proposed purpose is very similar to that of how the earliest of humans lived in their hunter-gatherer state, if you will recall from the first chapter.[64]

It would seem that a common thread among all of these examples is that a given thing's ultimate purpose is to *fulfill the function(s) that it is uniquely capable of fulfilling.* As such, in this view, the central purpose of modern humans is to fulfill what we alone can do. This would seem to refer to the use of our vastly superior intellect and heightened sense of emotional awareness. Our intellect is principally characterized by our ability to *reason*; that is, to make decisions about our actions using knowledge and evidence as to *why* they are the best decisions. While the decisions of animals, insects, and even plants are categorically based in instinct granted by a long evolutionary process, humans are instead able to critically reflect upon the consequences of a given action. This permits us to make an informed decision as to what course of action should be taken through the active consideration of the relevant situational factors.

To what end do we, or *should* we, direct our actions, though? This is where our other unique trait of emotional awareness comes in. We are able to reflect upon our own emotions *and* the emotions of others. As such, through our capacity for reason and our consequent capacity to act rationally, we therefore accrue *responsibility* for ensuring the emotional welfare of both ourselves and the people around us. This, of course, operates in addition to the more basic and longstanding purpose of ensuring the physical survival of both parties, as we have done since our inception as a species and as even far less intellectually-advanced species do.

Notably, decisions based on ensuring the survival of others in the early evolution of our species were arguably not *consciously* done and were therefore not of a purposeful or moral nature, persé. Even the late hunter-gatherers (and some subsequent generations of humans) who based their worldview in mythology founded their purpose and moral system merely in avoiding the bad consequences that would arise from certain actions. As such, for the most part they did not use traits such as advanced reason and empathy as their primary motivators in making decisions and thus did not attain an understanding of a deeper sense of purpose such as we are now able to.

Given our furthered rational, intellectual, and emotional capabilities since those times, emotional and physical welfare can therefore be combined into one ultimate responsibility: ensuring the well-being of ourselves and the other lives on the planet which we share. In this view, our broader purpose is therefore to act (using our reason and decision-making capabilities) in a way that fulfills our ultimate responsibility (ensuring the well-being of ourselves and other lives), which is granted to us by virtue of that which we are uniquely capable of doing (using our higher intellect and capacity for emotional awareness).

This is perhaps the most important point to consider: to paint a complete picture here, we must of course define what exactly "well-being" entails. For most of our history, well-being for homo sapiens (as well as most other life forms) has been characterized by "being in a state of pleasure". Pleasure, of course, has historically served as a natural indicator as to whether or not we are doing the correct things for the purpose of ensuring our survival.

Putting our hands in fire, of course, produces pain, and as such we have thankfully learned not to do that.

Consuming food (thereby nourishing yourself) produces pleasure, and as such we naturally learned to continue doing so in order to ensure our survival. Similarly, our long-term survival as a species has been predicated on the pleasure produced by sexual intercourse, leading to an instinctual drive to produce offspring.

From a Darwinian perspective, pain and pleasure serve as natural indicators to ensure that the process of natural selection runs smoothly. This is true even to the point that dominant animals that are at the top of the biological hierarchy have higher serotonin levels in the brain, which not only enhances pleasure but also allows the bearer to live longer.[65] This is a natural reward system for being the 'alpha'; in a sense, nature is aware that an alpha animal is likely to live longer and survive through increased strength, resourcefulness, and other related capabilities.

On the other hand, those that are at the lower end of the dominance and/or social hierarchy tend to have higher levels of cortisol (stress hormones) and lower levels of serotonin. Through our furthered intellectual and emotional capacities, however, it is evident that pleasure and being at the top of the biological hierarchy are not all that there is with regard to enhancing well-being and the human condition.[66]

Our enhanced understanding of ourselves and how we operate in the world around us has allowed us to understand that pleasure can often be a temporary and immediate sensation that can actually produce *negative* results in the long run. A simple example of this that comes to mind is the use of a drug such as heroin. Sure, one gets immense pleasure for a window of a few hours or so, but the long-term results of heroin use are quite obviously catastrophic, both mentally and physically. We are now also aware that pleasure does not necessarily have to be physical in nature; deeper mental processes can also bring about a sense of pleasure and contentment, such as the feeling of accomplishment when one completes a task or succeeds at a given goal.

It is important to note, however, that our emotional well-being and physical well-being are extraordinarily interdependent and one can often dictate the state of the other. Being lazy and inactive (although often pleasurable) not only serves as a detriment to our physical health, for instance, but can also contribute towards feelings of depression and anxiety. A further example is that constant mental worry can overload our bodies with the stress hormone cortisol, which can have terribly negative effects on the physical processes of our bodies.

Consequently, it is best for us to strive for a much deeper and wholesome sense of happiness if we wish to *truly* improve the well-being of both ourselves and those around us, now that we have a deeper sense of self-awareness and understanding. This is exactly why Aristotle wished for humans to strive for what he called '*Eudaimonia*'. As per its common translation from Greek, this term means 'happiness', although philosophers generally agree that the Ancient Greek philosophers (and especially Aristotle) instead refer to it in the sense of having a good indwelling spirit, furthering one's personal well-being, exercising good virtue, and living in a state of contemplation.[67]

Our unique capacity for rational thought has instilled in us an ability to avoid merely basing our actions on instinct like animals and like *we* used to do further back in our evolution. Instead, we are able to look towards the future and analyze both the immediate and long-term consequences of our actions. If we wish to live a meaningful life, then, we are naturally responsible for acting in such a way as to advance our *overall* well-being and that of others. Since we are the only living species on Earth that can consciously and effectively do this (and we are aware of our own mortality) this can be deemed as our central purpose.

This is, of course, just one conception of the concept of purpose, although its logical coherence and altruistic nature do allow it to serve as a powerful example. One major advantage of this conception of purpose is that it holds true independent of whether or not one believes in a deity or God. If you do believe in God, for instance, then this would naturally be interpreted as God purposefully having intended us to have these unique capabilities of intellectual superiority and emotional awareness through his creation process. If you do not believe in God and you are looking for your own sense of purpose, then there is no better place to start than looking at what you are uniquely capable of doing as part of the human species. This can then be further specified toward what you are most capable of doing as an individual, something which will be discussed in later chapters.

In this chapter we have looked our traditional understandings of the terms "meaning" and "purpose". Broadly speaking, while meaning seems to refer to the significance of life itself, purpose seems to refer to the reason life exists and the reasons we live for. A noteworthy conception of meaning is looking at the sheer rarity of life and the gratitude with which we should face being a way for the universe to understand itself. There is something to be said for being a part of something so vast, inspiring, and infinitely complex (yet paradoxically capable of sustaining us as fragile beings, for the time being). On the other hand, a great example of purpose is doing that which we are uniquely capable of doing, such as using our advanced intellect and emotional awareness to advance the human condition and the well-being of ourselves and others.

With this in mind, it is now time to begin your own journey to find your meaning and purpose. This chapter's exercise involves thinking about elementary definitions of meaning/purpose of your own as they pertain to your life. Don't worry if they are not perfect; that is exactly what you are here to work on throughout the course of this book. In light of what you have read thus far, write down whatever comes to mind when you think of the two terms. All that is necessary at the moment is just a basic framework of what you are personally trying to find when you think of pursuing meaning and purpose, and what it will have meant to you when you do discover them. Once you finish this, we will head to the next important step: knowing and understanding yourself.

<u>**Chapter 3 Reflection Questions**</u>

1.) What is it that you feel you are lacking in your life?

2.) What does the term 'meaning' mean to you, and what positive results would arise if you found your own sense of meaning in life (how do you imagine you would feel, for instance?)

3.) What does the term 'purpose' mean to you, and what positive results would arise if you found your own sense of purpose in life?

4

Who You Are... and Why

The Importance of Understanding Oneself

There remains a key problem in most Western educational systems that is seldom addressed, yet has profound effects upon our senses of meaning and purpose (or lack thereof) from a young age. This problem is that nearly everything that we learn pertains to things *outside* of ourselves; rarely are we taught how to look for answers from *within*. The ironic thing is that looking within through attempting to understand yourself can actually be amazingly beneficial with regard to your capabilities to learn about the outside world; in fact, it serves as the very foundation of learning. If students understand themselves better, they can set academic standards for themselves, figure out how they learn best, understand their motivations with regard to getting work done, properly explore their interests, and learn to improve upon their own weaknesses and foster their abilities.

Unsurprisingly, this same concept of understanding yourself will prove immensely valuable in discovering and subsequently acting upon your sense of meaning and purpose. Within the field of psychology, this phenomenon is referred to as *self-awareness*. Now this term appears quite easy to define. "Being aware of oneself" is probably the very first and simplest definition that comes to mind. However, it is important to avoid conflating self-awareness with self-consciousness. Self-consciousness refers to the mere awareness of one's own existence (think of a baby looking in the mirror and eventually learning that the person in the mirror is in fact their own self). Self-awareness, on the other hand, is perhaps equally important yet has a fundamentally deeper meaning.

Self-awareness broadly refers to observing the processes that occur in your own mind, and subsequently acting upon your observations as opposed to just experiencing your thought or emotive processes without any further reflection, as I would argue most people tend to do. This can be done in the form of reflecting upon your own needs, behaviors, habits, failures, successes, lived experiences, character, abilities, etc. so that you can act according to your own personal standards. Interestingly enough, becoming self-aware can also help you to *determine* those personal standards and values in the first place. I have come up with helpful way to illustrate the process of using self-awareness using five steps that have really helped both myself and my clients, and it goes as follows:

The Five Stages of Situational Self-Awareness

(1) Observation
(2) Establishment of Direct Cause
(3) Value Judgment
(4) Reflection
(5) Method of Change *or* Maintenance/Reinforcement

To demonstrate how this process works, let us take a relatively simple event and analyze it. Although this process can be used for nearly any type of occurrence in your life, for this example we will use an instance in which we are analyzing a particular emotional response:

(1) Observation: I angrily yelled at my partner today, causing her to leave the room in tears.

(2) Establishment of Direct Cause: My partner kept asking me to do things even though I was late for work.

(3) Value Judgment: Anger is not an emotion that enjoy feeling, and hurting others is something I want to avoid at all costs.

(4) Reflection: As per my value judgment of this event, I wish to avoid such events in the future. Upon further reflection, I probably got so angry because I was stressed out over being late for work. My partner was also running late, so I can see why she might have needed my help with what she was asking me for.

(5) Method of Change: I will talk to my partner about the event and we will work out a solution collaboratively. I think that getting things ready at night for the next day would be a huge benefit in case something like this were to ever happen again, and I should also set two alarms so that we don't wake up late. Instead of reacting angrily, which only made the problem worse, I will ensure to keep both of our best interests in mind and approach future problems in a level-headed and rational manner.

Interestingly enough, by merely categorizing this as a perceived negative event, we have established two important values of our own: being angry is not a good thing, and hurting others is something that is to be avoided. It is also important to note that this process does not have to be used for individual instances or events; it can also be used for observed repeated behaviours or even something as broad as your own character traits.

The regular use of this self-awareness process can help you to establish your macro-level values as they pertain to all aspects of your life, and of course, understanding our values plays a crucial role in the understanding of our meaning and purpose. Self-awareness tools like this one also help to create an element of accountability in your life. Instead of always saying "Oh, such and such happened to me" or "my emotions took over" as if you were not in control of the circumstances, it instead confers responsibility for your own actions, reactions, character traits, etc. and allows you to come up with your own solutions. As mentioned in the previous chapter, responsibility plays a *huge* role when one is trying to figure out one's purpose; having a purpose necessarily entails self-imposed responsibilities that you are morally required to fulfill as per your own standards.

Since any method through which you pursue your purpose is very likely to involve communicating and interacting with others (such as your occupation, for instance) a deep sense of self-awareness will also help you to be able to understand and empathize with *others*. As a result, interactions that you have with them can be mutually beneficial and based on a shared sense of understanding as to the goals of both parties.

Speaking of others, when it comes to broader elements of your life such as your character, the use of external opinions from others can also be immensely helpful. Taking into consideration how *others* feel about you can help you to understand how you appear to other people, and can also make you more self-aware of features that you may not have known about. This concept is outlined in an additional self-awareness tool that was created by psychologists Joseph Luft and Harrington Ingham called the **Johari Window**, which looks like this:[68]

Johari Window

	Known to self	Not known to self
Known to others	Arena	Blind Spot
Not Known to Others	Façade	Unknown

The creators of this tool initially intended it to be used by an individual seeking self-awareness and their peer(s). In the intended process of using this tool, both parties receive a list of 56 adjectives that they can use to describe the individual's behaviour, character, or motives, and they are organized into the above window afterwards. Each of the four boxes can be described as follows:

Arena: Traits that both the individual and their peers agree upon that describe the individual accurately.

Façade: Traits that the individual recognizes within themselves, but that others are not aware of. This can also indicate that the traits are perhaps untrue but the individual believes them to be true.

Blind Spot: Traits that the individual's peers use to describe the individual, but that the individual does not know about and/or agree with.

Unknown: Traits that neither the individual nor their peers are aware of. These could be unconscious elements of the individual's mind, unseen indicators of hidden potential, or things that the individual suppresses/denies and their peers are not aware of.

The Johari Window is an extremely useful tool since it takes into account the input of other people into one's self-awareness journey; something which may at first seem contradictory. However, this allows an individual to see the discrepancies that may exist between their perception of themselves and others' perception of them, and can elucidate some strengths that they did not know they had and/or some areas for improvement that they were not aware of.

The Power of Mindset: Our Beliefs and Biases

Perhaps one of the most fundamental elements of an individual's self-awareness journey is understanding their own basic belief system and any potential biases that they may hold. Belief systems and biases can be immensely powerful and life-changing – either negatively or positively. Belief systems and biases almost always operate deep within our subconscious and act as a filter which everything we experience passes through; one can think of them as the window through which you view the world. Belief systems have the power to alter our not only our psychology, but even our physiology.

Beliefs, generally defined, are assumptions that we hold to be true. One can believe that the Earth is flat, for instance, or that the moon landing never happened. On perhaps a more relatable level, one can believe that a certain amount of homework is detrimental to student success and well-being. These are all basic beliefs that pertain to one kind of thing or event. Then, there are beliefs that revered life coach Tony Robbins has described as "global" beliefs. Global beliefs are those that form one's belief system – a series of core beliefs that shape the way that we view the world and events that occur within it. In other words, your worldview and/or mindset is shaped by a set of foundational biases (although the word "bias" almost always has a negative connotation, healthily-formed biases can have *positive* effects).[69]

Two clear examples of global beliefs would be the belief that God exists, or that all people are inherently evil. Beliefs like these reshape the way that one sees the world, the events that occur within it, and everything that happens in their life; there is no escaping them since they apply in every instance that one might encounter. The power of both basic and global beliefs cannot be overstated. As Robbins writes, "With enough emotional intensity and repetition, our nervous systems experience something as real, even if it hasn't occurred yet."[70]

As a hypothetical example, think of a basic belief (even if it is loosely held, meaning it is essentially akin to a worry) that the elevator you are in is going to malfunction. What happens? Your heart rate goes up, you begin to feel nervous, your thoughts start racing with possibilities, and your body itches to get out as soon as possible. It triggers both an intense physical and mental response that varies depending on the strength of your belief. However, in 99.99% of cases, everything ends up going as per usual; the elevator reaches the destination, opens the doors, and you exit as if it were any other normal day.

If that is the power of a basic belief, imagine the power of a system of *global* beliefs built up over the course of your entire life. Here, one can begin to see the power that the increased knowledge we gained as a species (as illustrated in Chapter 2) could affect our senses of meaning and purpose. Just the one discovery of the Earth's ultimate fate alone (namely, being swallowed up by the Sun) could devastate an individual's belief system, causing them to believe that nothing is really worth it since we are inevitably doomed as a species in the end.

To further illustrate this concept, it is worth looking at two opposing types of mindsets that are each informed by differing global beliefs. In her seminal 2006 book titled "Mindset: The New Psychology of Success", Carol Dweck (a Stanford University psychology professor) highlighted the importance of our mindset in contributing to our achievement of success. Put simply, a mindset consists of a basic set of assumptions that we either implicitly or explicitly hold. This set of assumptions acts as a framework which informs the decisions that we make and the attitudes that we have in response to a given stimuli or challenge. Dweck proposes two central and opposing mindsets; namely, those that are *fixed* and those which are centered around *growth*.

A *fixed* mindset is one in which an individual believes that various traits (whether it be their character, intelligence, athletic capabilities, and/or moral compass) are static; that is, they are inherent and unchangeable in any significant way. This leads a person to attempt to strive merely to show that they have been born with superior qualities instead of striving for constant improvement. As such, not only are they disproportionately inclined to attempt to prove themselves to others, but they also will avoid failure at all costs, even to the point of denial. That is because in this mindset, any indication of failure is seen merely as a reflection of an unalterable trait that is permanently held by the individual. Repeated failures, then, are likely to be seen as an indication that they were merely dealt a bad hand from birth and will never succeed.[71]

A growth mindset, on the other hand, is one based upon the belief that these traits can be improved through investing time and effort into them. There is no inherent need, then, to prove oneself to other people because improvement is always possible. Those with a growth mindset see challenges and failures as opportunity for learning and improvement. Their mind automatically seeks solutions to problems and areas for improvement after failure. While everyone is inevitably given basic traits and qualities that they start out with, those with a growth mindset do not feel bound by them; rather, they merely see them as a foundation upon which to build.[72]

If not given sufficient examination through the process of self-awareness, these mindsets both work on a subconscious level of sorts since any decision we make or problem that we are faced with automatically goes through our mindset like a filter. Your response to any given stimuli is dictated by which of these mindsets you subscribe to. One can quite easily see how these two mindsets would not only affect peoples' lives and worldview, but also their sense of meaning and purpose in life. It is important to evaluate not only the empowering beliefs that you hold, but also the limiting beliefs that you hold by examining the references and evidence (or lack thereof) upon which you have built them up. This can help to eliminate any negative thought patterns and reinforcements in your head that have no basis in reality and merely serve to harm your sense of meaning and purpose.

Being aware of the beliefs that you hold is a massive part of becoming self-aware, and a necessary part of understanding your own meaning and purpose. Self-awareness is the key to understanding what it is exactly that you want in life and where you find meaning and purpose by re-evaluating the beliefs you hold, your behaviors, your lived experiences and how they have influenced you, etc.

It is very evident that self-awareness is an integral part of any individual's journey through life, but unfortunately it is not one that many pursue. With the knowledge you now have about self-awareness, let us look into the specific components of self-awareness that you will be asked to reflect upon with respect to your own life at the end of the upcoming chapter.

5

The Components of Self-Awareness

In this Chapter's exercises, you will be asked several questions pertaining to who you are so that you can become fully self-aware and are more prepared to consolidate your own sense of purpose in your life. As such, this chapter will provide you with incredibly useful information that you can use to help answer these questions. We are going to observe four major components of your life that, when recognized and reflected upon, will help you understand why you are the way that you are and will also help you to use this newfound understanding to inform your decisions moving forward into the future.

In many ways, as per the neuroplasticity of our brains (that is, the brain's ability to reorganize itself to adapt to new information), we are a summary of the experiences we have faced and how we have responded to those experiences. This new information (or stimuli) that we gather and our experiences can be broken down into four major components:

(1) Unconscious Foundations and Presuppositions
(2) Conscious and Supplementary Influences
(3) Positive Life Factors Thus Far
(4) Negative Life Factors Thus Far

To observe these components, we will start by delving into your unconscious mind. Sounds pretty scary, doesn't it? At the very least, I can assure you that it will be acutely enlightening.

(1) Unconscious Foundations, Presuppositions, and Supplementary Influences

The identification of the unconscious elements of your belief system and worldview is a pivotal tool through which you can analyze your biases with regard to your current conception of the meaning of life and your purpose. This can be an extremely challenging task, since, of course, your unconscious mind is beyond the reach of your conscious mind (at least *directly*). Now of course, you might be skeptical about the existence of your unconscious mind to begin with (as you probably have the right to be, since it is something relatively unobservable). The unconscious mind has been studied by psychologists such as Sigmund Freud and Carl Jung for centuries, and is generally characterized as consisting of the processes in the mind which occur automatically and cannot be consciously reflected upon while they are happening. However, they *can* later be deduced as *having happened* using retrospective evidence.

The diametric relationship between the conscious and unconscious mind is akin to the difference between voluntary and involuntary movements and bodily functions. It is a rather silly example, but let us take a brief look at the involuntary function of breathing. Chances are you do not consciously think about breathing all day, yet at the end of each day you can look back and say "Hey, the human body requires oxygen to survive, and we consume oxygen through regular breathing. I'm alive at the end of this wonderful day, so therefore I can deduce that I must have breathed regularly all day!" Ninety-nine percent of the time, breathing occurs unconsciously – you are not consciously aware of it happening, but your brain is making it happen nonetheless (and thank goodness!) While this is a more physically-oriented example, let us instead look at some unconscious mental processes that illustrate what the unconscious mind is capable of and get a glimpse of how it can impact both the way we perceive the world *and* our place within it.

One intriguing mental process that is based in our unconscious mind is the act of dreaming. Dreams have been an intriguing subject of close psychological study for centuries, and we still have yet to come to a full understanding of them. The interpretation of dreams has been attempted by psychologists like Sigmund Freud (who believed them to be expressions of unconscious desires) and Carl Jung (who believed that they are expressions of a collective unconscious amongst humanity), as well as countless other individuals who believe that their dreams are in some way significant to them. If there is one thing to be agreed upon with regard to dreams, it is that they are indeed an unconscious process.[73]

Dreams occur when we are sleeping, and we do not consciously create them (since, of course, we are in an unconscious state). Our dreams can often be extremely emotionally intense and complex, causing us to be puzzled if we wake up and are able to remember them. In other words, they can affect us when we are conscious/awake and reflect back upon them. What is interesting is that even if we do not instantly remember them, they can still affect us in quite substantial ways.

A rather comical example is an instance I can recall in which my partner and I woke up, and I noticed throughout the day that she was fairly irritable and inexplicably hostile towards me relative to most days, although I could not figure out why for the life of me. Upon asking her about it she said that she could not explain it either and was deeply apologetic. Later in the day, around 5pm, she said "Oh my God, I just remembered a dream I had last night!" Funnily enough, it was a dream in which I had apparently treated her very rudely. As it turns out, it seems that she had consciously acted out in a way that apparently reflected perceived unconscious events that never actually happened in reality.

According to most psychologists, dreaming is a phenomenon through which our unconscious interprets and processes through our experiences, often in a narrative format. Dreams can be a surprisingly intricate expression of a wide range of things including our fears, desires, emotional state, etc. If anything, it is widely agreed upon that they serve as strong evidence that the unconscious mind can be immensely powerful; anyone who has experienced a terrifying nightmare can certainly attest to this. Upon waking up from a nightmare you can even feel physiological symptoms of fear such as a vastly increased heartrate even though, in reality, nothing is happening; you were likely to be sound asleep in a comfortable and safe bed the entire time.

A second major mental phenomenon that is based in the unconscious mind is the concept of memory. Our memory is where we store our experiences with past events, facts, feelings, etc. Obviously our mind is not constantly perceiving these memories, or else we would have one heck of a chaotic situation in our heads. Instead, they are stored in an unconscious part of the brain where they can later be consciously accessed and retrieved when necessary. Amazingly enough, this unconscious 'storage unit' has been estimated to have a storage capacity equivalent to *one million gigabytes* of digital data, which is roughly *200 million* songs' worth of storage space.[74] Of course, we can draw upon memories to inform the decisions that we make (such as which route to take while driving, or what answer to write during an exam). However, our memories can also *unconsciously* inform the decisions that we make.

Imagine someone who, in their childhood, had a scary experience with a person dressed as a clown. In the future, they might very well have a fearful response whenever they see clowns again, even without consciously thinking of the very first experience that initially scared them. In other words, it is an automatic unconscious response. It is certainly a scary prospect, but by virtue of it having been too long since the first encounter, or them having been too young, or them having repressed the memory, they might not even be able to *consciously recall or remember* that the experience happened in the first place. Despite these factors it can still have an immense unconscious impact upon their 'worldview' and physiological responses when it comes to clowns.

On the other hand, *positively* perceived memories can also unconsciously effect our habits and conscious decisions. Imagine someone who had tried heroin at a party when they were a teenager. They might have experienced a level of physical pleasure that they previously did not think was possible. The individual then starts to seek out the drug throughout the next week, and engages in using heroin again. Eventually, this turns into a habit. Each time the individual subsequently uses heroin, however, they might not consciously think back to the previous times they used it and what they felt; instead, their physical and mental unconscious memories of using the drugs naturally associate pleasure with its use. While the individual might make the conscious decision to use the drug each time, it is their unconscious memories that subtly *influence* that decision.

Since everything we know and have experienced resides in our memory, all of our major beliefs and belief systems are substantiated by a series of references that are rooted in our unconscious, many of which were also created unconsciously. By reflecting upon our actions, behaviours, habits, and beliefs and associating them with a deduced cause (such as unconscious influences), we can learn to re-evaluate them and ensure that they are not only what we truly believe to be correct, but that they are beneficial to our lives.

At the end of this chapter, you will be asked to reflect upon your personal unconscious influences. These can be organized into three major groups, namely: **Sociocultural Influence**, **Familial Influence**, and **Sociodemographic Influence**. These are three kinds of unconscious influences that often impact the way we see the world without us even knowing it, unless, of course, we reflect upon them through the process of introspection. The three groups of influences can be described as follows:

Sociocultural Influence: This category of influence primarily has to do with the societal and cultural environment in which you were raised and have experienced life. This most often refers to elements of the country (or countries) in which you have lived, but can also be further specified to a region or community within a country. Sociocultural influences are derived from the *philosophical, political, legal,* and *cultural* foundations of the areas or political entities in which you have lived.

In Western countries, for instance, the philosophical traditions are likely to be heavily influenced by the Judeo-Christian religion, which outlines the values that are reflected in the domestic laws which you have (hopefully) conformed to throughout your life. In countries like these, the political system is likely to be democratic in nature, and the population composition is likely to be quite multicultural. Even if you do not think things like these have influenced you, in reality they inevitably *have* by virtue of you living within this system, conforming to it, having it shape your sociocultural worldview, and by virtue of it constituting the 'norm' in your perspective.

Familial Influence: This kind of influence primarily refers to the nature of your upbringing by your parents and/or caretakers. This can include things like parenting/caretaking styles (disciplinary and reward systems, for instance), values that you were taught to uphold, religious influences from those individuals, the nature of the relationship between family members, whether or not you were an only child, and numerous other factors pertaining to unconscious influences from the people within your household or living environment.

Sociodemographic Influence: This type of influence refers to factors surrounding things like your ethnicity, gender, sexuality, your family's economic status, your neighbourhood, etc. The circumstances surrounding features of ourselves and the availability of resources dictate the way in which we see the world – take the earlier example of a poorer person likely being more pessimistic about life than a richer person, for instance. These factors act as an unconscious lens through which we see the world, and are extremely important to consider.

(2) Conscious and Supplementary Influences

In addition to unconscious influences that inevitably affect our worldview, we also experience *conscious* influences that we are usually well aware of, whether that is because we actively chose to engage with them or we were old enough to be able to acknowledge and reflect upon them at the time they occurred. Since conscious influences are significantly easier to understand and observe, we will go straight into the three major groups that they are comprised of: **External & Situational Influence, Educational Influence,** and **Biological & Psychological Influence**.

External & Situational Influence: This type of influence refers to things that are extracurricular in nature and usually pertain to activities that you engaged in of your own choice. This can refer to a broad spectrum of things, with some examples being: any books you have read outside of school, movies you have watched, the types of Youtube videos you have watched, the extent to which you use social media, video games, music, athletic activities/sports, whether or not you have used any drugs, etc. Essentially, these influences constitute anything that you have actively chosen to engage in (outside of mandated things such as school) that has shifted or enhanced your perspective on your life and/or the world around you.

Educational Influence: This one is relatively obvious; it refers to influences derived from any educational settings that you have experienced. Important factors to consider here are how many educational institutions you attended, the quality of your education, your performance in school, the types of things that you learned/studied, the nature of your education (whether you went to a secular, religious, or private school, for instance), as well as your social status within those institutions, defining occurrences and events, and the kinds of social interaction you had with others during your education.

Biological & Psychological Influence: Biological influences can include things like your race and ethnicity, but more specifically include things like your perceived aesthetic appearance, fitness level, any physical disabilities and/or health problems you may have, etc. Biology also determines your psychological influences, which can include things like any diagnosed mental health problems/disorders that you have (such as a tendency toward depression or anxiety, for instance). These physical and mental attributes can all have immense influence on the way that you perceive the world around you and are extremely important to take into consideration when trying to find meaning and your purpose in life.

(3) Positive Life Factors Thus Far

In addition to examining your influences, taking into consideration the things that you consider to be positive about your life can help to indicate what things you value and what things you should continue to pursue and improve upon. It can also help you to determine your strengths, which is a key part of being able to figure out your purpose since it usually involves the pursuit and fulfillment of things that you excel at and value. If possible, I would highly recommend that you make use of the principles described earlier in the Johari Window by having a truthful close friend or partner join in on this activity to elucidate some of your *blind spots*; that is, positive features that they would honestly describe you as that you might not have otherwise seen.

There are five central things that you will be asked to list and reflect on with regard to positive life factors, including: **Accomplishments**, **Positive Character Traits**, **Skills/Abilities**, **Areas of Specialty**, and **Good Habits**. It will be helpful to know what these entail before attempting to identify your own. These life factors can be broadly described as follows:

Accomplishments: This area of course refers to major life events that you consider to be accomplishments that you have personally achieved and that fulfilled a particular goal of yours. When considering this life area, try to think of things that you have expended a substantive amount of effort to achieve and things that you are proud of yourself for having accomplished. Common examples include getting your high school diploma or a college/university degree, reaching a certain level of achievement in a sport, completing a personal project, being hired at a job you worked hard to get, etc.

Good Character Traits: This merely refers to positive adjectives that you would use to describe yourself. Examples would include descriptors like *humble*, *determined*, *hard-working*, *dependable*, etc. You should be able to come up with at least ten of these. The more you have, the more complete of a picture you can paint of yourself and the qualities you regard as being valuable.

Skills/Abilities: This section refers to *specific* things that you believe yourself to have considerable skill/ability with. In other words, these are particular things that you excel at or consider yourself to be "above average" in doing. Examples would include things like critical thinking, cooking, writing, etc.

Areas of Specialty: As opposed to specific skills, this section instead refers to broader areas that you are proficient in or have a notable level of expertise with. Looking at most of your skills/abilities, what broader categories do they fall into? Examples of these include academia, fitness, business, music, craftsmanship, art, etc.

Good Habits: Good habits refer to things that you do regularly (usually daily) that improve the quality of your life and/or the quality of the lives around you. Examples would include going to the gym, getting a good amount of sleep, eating healthily, making food for your significant other, etc.

(4) Negative Life Factors Thus Far

Observing the negative factors in your life can be an extremely challenging process, and one that requires a high level of self-awareness and humility. No one is perfect – but to become our best selves and understand our meaning and purpose, we must first be able to recognize not only the areas that we *can* improve upon, but also those we think we either *want* to improve upon or feel we *should* improve upon. Making these judgments not only improves your self-awareness and indicates areas that you can pursue improvement in, but it can also make significant indications as to the nature of your sense of meaning and purpose.

If I feel that my sleep schedule is poor and needs improvement for the sake of my health, for instance, that shows that I *value* taking care of myself – which is therefore a small aspect of my broader purpose (perhaps I might recognize that taking care of myself allows me to better take care of the ones I love, for example). Recognizing these negative life factors also gives you a direction to move in with regard to several areas of your life, and a deeply-held reason for doing so.

Again, and perhaps more importantly than with positive life factors, it is immensely helpful to have an honest close friend or partner help you with your blind spots. Be sure to accept their opinions as an attempt to help you with the things you are unable to see and not as criticisms; this itself is a key part of being self-aware. If someone is willing to help you with this exercise, chances are that they are merely listing areas for improvement that they know will help you; it serves as newfound knowledge, which you should be thankful for. With regard to negative life factors, we will be looking at five major areas: **Failures**, **Negative Character Traits**, **Lacking Skills**, **Areas for Improvement**, and **Negative Habits**.

Failures: These refer to major negative events or occurrences in which you perceive yourself to have most (if not all) of the responsibility for allowing or causing to happen. It is important to keep in mind that these only constitute events that are within what author Stephen Covey calls your "Sphere of Influence" – things that you reasonably had control over. Attributing blame to yourself for negative events that you had little to no control over (such as a family member getting hurt by someone when you were not around) is immensely unhealthy and unreasonable. Failures are instead major events in your life that you positively know you *could have* reasonably avoided had you invested the proper care, time, or effort.

Examples of failures would include losing a job you were not very committed to, failing to complete a personal project because you lost motivation, dropping out of school, major incidents in which you failed to uphold your moral code (cheating on a spouse, for instance), etc. It is important to be very honest with yourself; your Foundational Document is yours alone and will be able to impact your life more positively the more truthful and self-aware you are.

Negative Character Traits: These refer to negative adjectives that you would use to describe yourself. These traits should in some way be perceived by you as being harmful to yourself and/or those around you. Examples include being *overly anxious, reckless, lazy, judgmental,* etc. This should not be seen as an open opportunity to harshly criticize or pity yourself, but rather to indicate some areas for improvement with regard to your character and habits. Again, aim for ten or more adjectives since these serve as self-developed indications as to what you should pursue in the future and therefore will reveal a significant part of your purpose moving forward.

Lacking Skills: These are specific skills/abilities that you lack, but that you would either *like* to have or think you *should* be proficient in for any given reason. Examples include understanding an additional language, being able to make healthy food for yourself or your family, etc.

Areas for Improvement: These include broader areas or categories of knowledge that you do not feel yourself to be proficient in despite the fact that you wish to be or feel that you should be. In other words, you know that they will be beneficial to you and/or others in some way. Examples include social skills, academic subjects, human psychology, etc.

Negative Habits: These are of course regular actions or behaviours that you engage in, but that impact your life (or the lives of others) in a negative manner. Examples include doing drugs, the overuse of social media, staying inside too often, having a poor sleep schedule, eating unhealthy food, etc.

It is important that when answering this chapter's questions about unconscious and conscious influences and positive/negative life factors, you not only write down all of the influences you can think of, but also think about *how these may affect your sense of meaning, purpose, worldview, and quality of life* in your head as you go along. Remember to refer back to the respective descriptions and examples of the influences if you are stuck on answering a question pertaining to a particular type of influence.

Chapter 5 Reflection Questions

Unconscious Influences

1.) List all of the potential Sociocultural Influences that might have had an impact on you.

2.) List all of the potential Familial Influences that might have had an impact on you.

3.) List all of the Sociodemographic Influences that might have had an impact on you.

Conscious Influences

1.) List all of the External Influences that have had an impact on you.

2.) List all of the Educational Influences that have had an impact on you.

3.) List all of the Biological/Psychological Influences that have had an impact on you.

Positive Life Factors Thus Far

1.) What major accomplishments have you achieved in your life?

2.) What are some good character traits that you have?

3.) What skills do you have?

4.) What are your areas of specialty?

5.) What good habits do you have in your daily and/or weekly life?

Negative Life Factors Thus Far (Be Honest!)

1.) What are some major failures that you have experienced in your life?

2.) What are some bad character traits that you have?

3.) What specific things do you lack skill with that you think you *should* improve upon?

4.) What broader areas of life do you think you could improve upon?

5.) What bad habits do you have in your daily life?

6

Your Philosophical Foundations

By now you are likely to have a much clearer and well-defined idea of both who you are and how you have become who you currently are. In the last chapter, you made numerous value judgments with regard to your influences and life factors. In other words, you categorized influences and life factors as either being good or bad for both you and the people who come into contact with you. These value judgments are certainly important, as they indicate the direction that you believe your life *should* go in and what directions you should *avoid*. However, although the previous chapter likely encouraged you to foster a sense of self-awareness at a deeper and more extensive level than anything you have done before (and you probably gained more insight because of it), it is worthy to note that you have probably done something similar to this process before, but on a much smaller scale with particular instances that you have encountered.

For example, if you have had trouble with your sleep schedule in the past, you have probably recognized this fact one morning when you woke up extremely tired, groggy, and unmotivated. Yet, the cycle probably did not abruptly end. Instead, you likely kept going to bed late because you made several situational *micro-level* value judgments that were rooted in the immediate present late at night. For example, watching the next episode of a Netflix show each night might have been more valuable to you at the time then getting the proper sleep you needed to perform properly the next day. Yet retrospectively, you might have still made the *foundational macro-level* value judgment that getting enough sleep is more important to your well-being than binging episodes of a show on Netflix. It is this exact value judgment discrepancy that characterizes the lives of so many people worldwide.

This kind of discrepancy ultimately arises from a lack of *conviction*. A conviction is a type of belief that is so strongly held that it is nearly inseparable from the individual who holds it. Convictions can further be described as thoughts that are backed up by a system of beliefs and are further substantiated by evidence that supports those beliefs. When it comes to foundational macro-level value judgments that apply in all circumstances, one needs to have a *conviction* that they do indeed always apply. Convictions arise from a sense of meaning and purpose with regard to a certain situation.

In order for convictions to do their job (that is, ensure that you abide by your macro-level values), they need to be grounded in an individual's *core philosophy*. It is this exact phenomenon that so many people in the Western world are lacking, either through having given up on the concept altogether or by determining that they do not need one to get by. Therefore, even if an individual *does* decide to hold values that they wish to abide by, they are often loosely held and seldom followed because they are not *grounded* in anything that is substantive.

Earlier we discussed the concept of philosophy as a certain form of academic study that is motivated by the love (or *philos*) of wisdom (or *sophia*). In this context, we are discussing philosophy as a system of thought about the fundamental nature of reality and existence that is held dear to an individual. This pertains to two of the five central branches of philosophy, namely *Epistemology* (the study of knowledge) and *Metaphysics* (the study of the nature of reality). As such, there are two centrally linked questions that one needs to look at when attempting to establish their own core philosophy: (1) "What is the nature of reality?" and (2) "To what extent are we able to know about that nature?" Now, these questions might sound intense, but rest assured that this problem can be looked in quite a simple yet effective way.

Thanks to our extensive understanding of science (and most particularly astronomy), we now know that the universe began in a process called the "big bang" and that our universe has been accelerating and expanding outward ever since. For our purposes, finding our conception of the nature of reality is as 'simple' as determining how the creation of our universe (the big bang) occurred in the first place. Since our understanding of science cannot yet determine a concrete answer for this question, we are limited to holding *beliefs* about the nature of our existence.

Insofar as our current understanding extends, we are limited to two competing beliefs in attempting to explain our existence: either the universe was created purposefully, or it happened randomly/by chance. While the former option denotes the existence of some sort of metaphysical phenomenon or being ("metaphysical" in this sense meaning beyond our current scientific understanding) that intentionally created the universe, the latter entails the *lack* of a metaphysical creator. The positions that you can take with regard to this problem can be further distinguished into three broad schools of thought or metaphysical worldviews:

Theism: Theism is simply defined by the Oxford Dictionary as the "Belief in the existence of a god or gods, specifically of a creator who intervenes in the universe."[75]

Atheism: The Oxford Dictionary defines atheism as the "Disbelief or lack of belief in the existence of God or gods."[76]

Agnosticism: Agnosticism can be seen as a kind of 'middle ground' between the former two positions, and is defined as "[The belief] …that nothing is known or can be known of the existence or nature of God."[77]

While there are numerous sub-classifications of each one of these positions, for our purposes it is only necessary to know which position you broadly categorize yourself as being an adherent of. This discernment is extraordinarily important for establishing meaning, as it serves as the foundation of quite literally all of existence and as such serves as the quintessential *source* of meaning on both a personal and foundational level. It is important to note that, contrary to popular belief, establishing a consolidated sense of meaning *is* possible with all three of these options.

For theists, meaning (or special significance) is derived from the fact that the universe and human beings, by extension, were created by one or more beings that are beyond our comprehension. For atheists and agnostics, both of whom lack an active belief in God(s), meaning can be derived from phenomena such as the extreme rarity of life, our immense fortune to be able to explore and understand that from which we are created (the universe), and our fortune to be able to have evolved with emotional sentience so we can feel things like happiness and love (and have the capacity to help others feel those things as well). If you will remember, all of these conceptions of meaning were discussed in great detail in Chapter 3.

Admittedly, there are some noteworthy benefits to being a theist with respect to finding meaning and purpose. First is the fact that the majority of humanity held a common belief in God(s) for millennia and they are reflected in our traditions and political systems. However, this conception does comes at the price of being all the more painful when these beliefs are cast into doubt by events, discoveries, and demographic/political changes such as those that we discussed in Chapter 2. Secondly, meaning is inherently obvious if you are a theist. Believing in a metaphysical being beyond our comprehension that created the universe with you in mind provides instant special significance to one's life.

Finally, theistic beliefs that are associated with a particular religion provide a natural sense of purpose as well, since they are grounded in doctrines that indicate exactly what the human race's purpose is and how it can be achieved (usually through aligning oneself most closely with God's will, as outlined in the holy texts). These three reasons are probably a large part of why studies frequently show that religious individuals are usually happier, have a greater level of life satisfaction, have a higher sense of subjective psychological well-being, and have a clearer sense of meaning in their lives.[78]

One possible issue here, however, is that you might find yourself eventually disagreeing with some of the outlined purposes and moral entailments of your religion due to the reasons outlined in Chapter 2. This is natural, though, given that the holy texts were written by humans, none of whom are perfect, and done so merely under the *inspiration* of God (and thus they are not immune to scientific and moral error).

Keep in mind that if one finds themselves unable to agree with the tenets of a given religion, this does not automatically preclude the possibility of believing in a deity if you find theism to be intellectually plausible; one can believe in a creator without being tied to a particular religious view of that creator. Again, all of this is not to say that atheists and agnostics cannot find meaning and purpose, but instead that they might merely have to think a bit harder about their own conception of these terms since they are not automatically granted to them by virtue of their existential belief system.

This chapter's questions will ask you to reflect upon which one of the three aforementioned camps you fall into with regard to your existential beliefs, and what that means to you. Chances are, you are already well aware of which one you belong to, since questions of an existential nature are very hard to escape when you are a human being who is capable of sentience and philosophical thought. If you are unsure, go with the one that you feel deep down that you believe in as per your experiences and reflections thus far. If you are absolutely stuck and think that there is an exact 50/50 chance of each being the case (that is, the existence and nonexistence of god or gods), that naturally means you would be classified as an Agnostic.

The core philosophical camp that you categorize yourself as belonging to has a profound effect on one's life and worldview and also serves as a critical foundation for your sense of meaning. It also affects your sense of purpose through indicating the fundamental *source* of your morals and ethics, which will be discussed further in the upcoming chapter.

Chapter 6 Reflection Questions

Your Core Philosophy

1.) What philosophical worldview do you most strongly identify with: Theism, Atheism, or Agnosticism? Why?

2.) What special significance does (or *can*) life have under this worldview?

7

Establishing a Moral and Ethical System

The Competing Foundations of Morality

Morality and ethics are hotly debated topics worldwide, and for good reason. These two concepts act as guidelines that govern our actions, and can be instituted in various forms ranging from written laws that govern billions of people to personal codes that are self-imposed by an individual. Morality proves to be quite difficult to define given its very personal nature, but philosophers James and Stuart Rachels established a noteworthy 'minimum conception of morality' in an attempt to ensure that we at least have a basic definition of morality that can apply to most (if not all) people.

This minimum conception of morality is described as follows: "Morality is, at the very least, the effort to guide one's conduct by reason – that is, to do what there are the best reasons for doing – while giving equal weight to the interests of each individual affected by one's decision."[79] As per this definition, morality is therefore a very personal exercise, but can become more of a collective exercise if a given group of people share a common belief system.

As discussed in Chapter 2, a given democratic country's laws typically reflect that country's philosophical traditions combined with an average result of the current population's moral intuitions. It is worthy to note that these intuitions are capable both of reflecting and responding to demographic shifts within that population through the voting/legislative process. While these moral expressions can be followed by the population due to a mere fear of penalties (such as fines or prison time), each individual also maintains their own personal and/or communal morals which they attempt to uphold while operating within their country's political and legal system.

What many fail to actively consider, however, is the *foundational nature* and *source* of morality, which is based in one's core philosophy of life. These two things are discernable through determining which view of morality you adhere to: either *Objective* or *Subjective* morality. Simply explained, an *objective* view of morality regards morals as being absolute, definite, objective, and universally applicable in nature. A *subjective* view of morality, on the other hand, regards morals as being indeterminate, indefinite, and not inherent in objective reality, but rather as a creation of human beings. The view that you take with regard to morals being objective or subjective in nature is immensely influential and directly relates to your sense of purpose. There are two primary reasons why the proper distinction between the two perspectives of morality is so important:

(1) They Underpin the Nature and Purpose of Morality

Objective View: If morality is objective in nature, our purpose as humans is to align our actions with foundational moral truths that are grounded in reality and are therefore universally applicable. In this view, we have an objective duty as conscious, reflective, and self-aware entities to adhere to these indisputable moral principles and fulfill them through the use of our own individual capabilities insofar as we are able to.

Subjective View: If morality is subjective in nature, morality is largely indeterminate and moral systems are established and adhered to only insofar as they prove to be socioculturally, politically, and psychologically useful in establishing order, peace, and well-being for living beings that reside within a given geographical and/or political entity.

(2) They Indicate the Source of Morality

Objective View: If morality is objective, moral truths are, insofar as our scientific knowledge extends, grounded upon metaphysical foundations that not only allow for their existence, but also insist, recommend, and/or desire that humans adhere to them.

What is interesting about this perspective of morality is that truly objective foundations of morality have yet to be found by humankind through any demonstrable method. Therefore, objective sources of morality (if they are to exist), must exist outside of the explored world. In any tangible sense, this would mean these sources are beyond our current knowledge, thereby making them a part of metaphysical phenomena.

This idea is further explored by Canadian clinical psychologist and Professor Jordan B. Peterson in his book titled *Maps of Meaning*. Peterson describes the world around us as having a sort of dualistic nature (which is reflected in the unique functions of the left and right hemispheres of our brain) comprised of what *can* exist as per conscious decisions being made, and what merely *does* exist:

The world can be validly construed as forum for action, or as place of things.

The former manner of interpretation – more primordial, and less clearly understood – finds its expression in the arts or humanities, in ritual, drama, literature, and mythology. The world as forum for action is a place of value, a place where all things have meaning. This meaning, which is shaped as a consequence of social interaction, is implication for action, or – at a higher level of analysis – implication for the configuration of the interpretive schema that produces or guides action.

The latter manner of interpretation – the world as place of things – finds its formal expression in the methods and theories of science. Science allows for increasingly precise determination of the consensually-validatable properties of things, and for efficient utilization of precisely-determined things as tools (once the direction such use is to take has been determined, through application of more fundamental narrative processes).[80]

In other words, the human capacity for conscious decision-making that guides our actions opens up a new domain in terms of the way reality functions. On the one hand, we have that which merely exists (what Peterson calls a place of things) which is governed by natural laws, most of which we have a near-complete understanding of. On the other hand, we have what *can* exist as per human decisions (a forum for action). Naturally, this leads our reflective minds to question the way that things *should* be since, in many ways, we have the power to shape the future through our actions. In the objective view of morality, then, there is a definite and indisputable way that things should be that is independent of human thought.

However, insofar as human exploration and knowledge goes as per the scientific method, the cosmos (or the universe) merely *is*; it simply *exists*. Aside from natural laws that govern the way things have operated and continue to operate, such as gravity, there is not yet any objective nor provable basis to for found for normative notions (that is, foundational scientific evidence for the way that things *should* be). For this to be the case, there must be something metaphysical which overtly dictates a preferred sequence of events or actions taken by humans.

Furthermore, the extension of normative notions to the behavior of human beings by this metaphysical entity would (a) Indicate its recognition of the free will of humans and (b) Prove that it has an awareness of and sense of preference as to how humans behave, thereby indicating that the choices of humans are in some way consequential to it. All of this necessitates that this entity must in some way have a personal nature since it: has a will of its own, has the capacity to be affected by human decisions (if only slightly), and it has expressed or unexpressed preferences as to which decisions humans should make. For this reason, the objective view of morality is almost always associated with a core philosophy based in theism (the belief in a god or gods), since a deity is the only conceivable metaphysical phenomenon capable of making such distinctions *and* having the power to establish (and possibly enforce) an objective morality.

Subjective View: If morality is subjective, morality is socioculturally constructed and ideally agreed upon by groups of humans, whose long evolution has either preferred or necessitated primitive forms of morality for the purpose of group/species survival. This morality has since become increasingly complex, which reflects the increase in complexity of its societal and political systems and the ever-expanding human ability to use reason to make decisions.

This evolutionary foundation of subjective morality is supported by the available literature, since much of it shows that even more primitive animals often engage in 'moral' actions such as mutually beneficial and fair play.[81] For instance, bigger rats will often allow smaller rats to win in a play fight so that the smaller rat does not get discouraged.[82] Examples like these demonstrate a primitive sense of morality among animals that, in the case of humans, has grown increasingly complex over a period of evolution spanning hundreds of thousands of years.

Since people often get them confused, it is worthy to note that in this context, subjective morality is to be considered as distinct from the concept of *moral relativism*. A moral relativist position would advocate that morality is *relative* to different groups of people and/or cultures. In other words, different groups of people can have different moral beliefs and still be 'correct' since those morals apply equally to both groups based on their distinct histories, cultural differences, political differences, or other factors. One can see, then, that moral relativism is more of its own sub-classification under the larger conceptual umbrella of subjective morality, but it does not constitute subjective morality itself. On the contrary, the end goal of subjective morality might be closer to trying to establish a universal set of moral standards that *all* humans can agree upon at a worldwide level, or *should* agree upon based on the principles of reason.

Despite this, the subjective view of morality still does maintain that there is no objective/metaphysical set of moral standards that exist independently of human construction. Interestingly, this does not preclude the possibility of their being a god; it merely means that the god does not interfere in the affairs of humans and/or has no vested interest in how they act (a position that can be considered similar to that of *deism*). Since the most common conceptions of god ascribe Him with a personal nature that has concern for how humans act, it is easy to see why the subjective view of morality is more common with those who subscribe to atheistic/agnostic worldviews.

As you may be able to tell, these views of morality each have their own set of advantages and disadvantages, which is perhaps one of the many reasons why they are so fiercely contested in both academic and political spheres. The following two pages consist of two tables that concisely outline some of the advantages and disadvantages of each respective view of morality. Be sure to take the listed factors into account when establishing and consolidating your own opinion on these two perspectives of morality, in addition to considering the nature of the core philosophy or metaphysical worldview that you identified with in the previous chapter.

Advantages of the Two Moral Perspectives

Objective	Subjective
(1) Moral truths exist and everyone is held accountable by this very fact.	**(1)** Morality is more capable of evolving with time and in light of changing circumstances.
(2) Objectivity allows for order and universal coherence & consistency.	**(2)** Morals are more easily discoverable and grounded since we create and systematize them.
(3) Acting morally is objectively preferable, meaning there can be no dispute nor uncertainty.	**(3)** Subjectivity is able to account for sociocultural differences and is democratic in nature.

Disadvantages of the Two Moral Perspectives

Objective	Subjective
(1) There is a lower capacity for change and evolution with time. **(2)** Morals are not easily located nor synthesized unless revealed to us by that which established them. If not overtly revealed to us, this can lead to competing claims. **(3)** People may follow these objective morals out of fear or expectation of consequences instead of for altruistic or truly 'moral' reasons.	**(1)** Morals have no objective basis, meaning they are not necessarily true. **(2)** Moral relativism can be rampant, leading to chaos, a lack of consistency, and collective disagreement. **(3)** Accountability to uphold morals and motivation is more limited. **(4)** Morals are mainly grounded in utility and do not constitute morality as it is traditionally conceived.

Moral Conscious-Unconscious Alignment

It is important to note that when considering your moral perspective (and further specifying its entailments in the next chapter), you should also take into consideration the effects of your unconscious influences that we previously discussed. In other words, you need to *align* your unconscious influences and your conscious moral reflections in some significant way. If there is too great a discrepancy between the two (which can be termed as a *major existential discrepancy*), this can lead to existential and emotional crises of many forms, and perhaps most significantly a crisis of meaning.

On a collective level, this process is evidently happening within the Western world. The West's 'collective unconscious' (expressed through the philosophical foundation of Christianity in its laws, political systems, moral systems, etc.) has been steadily eroded by 'conscious reflections' (our increase in scientific knowledge, openness to widespread immigration, engagement in the economic system of capitalism, etc.) as it has evolved.

Similar crises can also be observed at the level of the individual. As we grow older, our belief systems usually evolve along with us, often causing us to supplant old beliefs in favor of others. In moderation, this can of course be a healthy and constructive process with benefits of numerous kinds. However, when a foundational unconscious belief *system* is eroded, this can often have catastrophic effects from which it becomes immensely difficult to recover.

The eroding of one's foundational belief system can very much be construed as a great *loss*; you either suddenly or gradually begin to lack something of the utmost foundational importance which you once had to guide you. As such, one is likely to undergo a process of grieving for that loss that bears resemblance to the stages of grief when one loses a close relative or gets diagnosed with a terminal illness, for instance. According to the Kübler-Ross model, the five stages of grief are Denial, Anger, Bargaining, Depression, and Acceptance.[83] One's crisis of meaning might follow a very similar pattern in that they might:

1.) Deny or attempt to disregard the new knowledge that they have acquired that casts their belief system into doubt.

2.) Eventually yield to the new knowledge out of intellectual necessity and get angry that their core belief system is not as true as they once believed (and possibly resent those who impressed it upon them in the first place).

3.) Begin an attempt to bargain or reconcile their former belief system with their new one (or lack thereof). If this fails, then:

4.) Become depressed, leading one to ask questions such as "Has my whole life been a lie? What is the purpose of my life? Why should I do anything at all? Is there any actual meaning in life? Do I even have a true purpose?" If these questions cannot be answered properly, then they will likely:

5.) Finally accept the state that they are in out of a sense that they will never escape it or find out the truth. This feeling can express itself in varying ways, including foregoing morality altogether and living recklessly, pursuing hedonistic desires, failing to do anything worthwhile with their life out of a sense that nothing is worth the effort, etc., all of which further the crisis since they are likely to violate the tenets of the their own unconscious influences.

One can see, then, that the bargaining and reconciliation process (Stage 3) is of the utmost importance. If this process is not conducted correctly, then everything can fall apart and a resolution will not be reached.

A prime example of this process is an individual who was raised in a Christian household and regularly attended church as a child, but later began to lose his/her faith as they learned more about science and the horrors of religious conflict. Having based the foundation of their life upon a sense of meaning and purpose grounded in the tenets Christianity, it becomes extraordinarily difficult to establish a new core philosophy. Not only that, but their unconscious inevitably remains attached to the teachings of the religion, including its moral guidelines. A conflict arises between their unconscious beliefs (which they may even attempt and fail to consciously deny) and their more recent conscious actions, which can express itself in terms of emotional damage and existential nihilism, if even moderately.

This can just as easily happen to someone who was raised in an agnostic/atheist household as well. For the most part (with the exception of those who were raised in an abusive or otherwise harmful environment), individuals tend to be relatively optimistic in their childhood because everything is about that which is immediate; life is about the next treat, the next fun event, the next exciting game. As we grow older, we become more emotionally and intellectually aware. We are able to reflect on the world at a deeper philosophical level and as such we understand realities that are incompatible (or even contrary to) our unconscious foundations. For those who grow up in agnostic/atheist environments, this can even be expressed in the form of realizing that the morals their caregivers instilled with them are not based in anything objective or that is tangible in the real world.

No matter your situation with regard to a crisis of this sort (even if you merely find your sense of meaning and/or purpose to be shaky), the key is to be found in the alignment and reconciliation of the conscious and unconscious mind. This is an extremely difficult and challenging process, which is why crises of this sort are so common in today's world both collectively and among individuals. If you feel you have lost your sense of meaning and/or purpose, it is key that you reflect back to before this loss occurred, even if this entails going as far back as your childhood when existential notions were likely of little to no consequence given your limited ability to think deeply about them. It is probable that your sense of meaning and purpose was instilled in you by your parents and/or caregivers, and it is important to reconcile these unconscious foundations with the conscious influences that you have since established.

With regard to the example given earlier, for instance (going from Theism to Atheism or Agnosticism, or even just having a less strong belief in God), one might have been raised in a more fundamentalist light with strict teachings about the Bible. Upon developing the capacity for critical reflection of the Bible's teachings, one might realize that much of the moral system developed in the Old Testament conflicts with their basic moral intuitions (for instance, advocating for the genocide of those who lived in the Amalek nation, encouraging slaves to submit to their masters and women to submit to their husbands, the use of stoning as a punishment for rebellious children, etc.)

A useful method of reconciliation in this case, then, would be to recognize that the Bible was written by man and that it was merely created under the *inspiration* of God, and therefore has room for some moral and scientific error but provides general guidelines that have, for the most part, become actualized in much of Western society. The recognition that Jesus' teachings supplant and/or revise those of the Old Testament's could also serve as being useful, as most modern Christians adhere mostly to the New Testament (which, while not perfect, is decidedly less morally objectionable).

In other words, your unconscious mind could be appeased by bringing the positive underlying entailments of your religion's teachings (that you know benefit your life) forward with you, that way you are retaining its core essence even if your belief in God itself has faltered. If this is indeed your situation, keep in mind that the West's political systems are philosophically based in Christianity, and by adhering to the laws of your country you are, in effect, living in correspondence with your unconscious.

For agnostics/atheists who eventually grow up to believe that their moral system has no substantive foundation in reality, it might be worthy to note the utility of moral systems and the viability of subjective morality as we discussed previously. Alternatively, one could realize that morality that is based on religious tenets often inspires people to act morally merely out of the fear of consequences. Instead, you could realize that your moral actions have been (and can continue to be) out of a true sense of altruism given the lack of metaphysical consequence for acting against a given set of morals (such as eternal punishment in the afterlife). In this situation, one could move forward using reason to help to establish a universal system of morality that strives toward the thriving of humanity.

It is important to note that these are merely two examples of reconciliation from opposite sides of the philosophical spectrum. The human population's crises of meaning are arguably much too diverse for any work to cover the alignment process in specific detail for each type of situation, but these examples should give you a general idea of how one should approach the reconciliation of unconscious influences and conscious reflections if necessary.

Notably, this process should not be mistaken with the notion that you should inevitably *return* to your unconscious foundations, but rather that you should recognize them (as you did in the last chapter) and reconcile them with your current beliefs in some substantive way so that a conflict is not brewing inside you. This chapter's reflection questions will later help you to work this process through in more detail.

The Ethical Parallel

Interestingly enough, the path that we have taken thus far in discovering your moral and ethical system has followed a logical progression that mirrors that which is found in the scholarly study of ethics as a whole. With regard to the ethics, there are three major academic fields of study: *Metaethics*, *Normative Ethics*, and *Applied Ethics*. These areas of study can each be described as follows:

1.) *Metaethics*: Concerns the theoretical meaning and reference of moral propositions, and how their truth values (if any) can be determined. In other words, it is the very study of the concept and nature of ethics itself.

2.) *Normative Ethics*: Concerns the practical means of determining a moral course of action. In other words, it is the study of how one can determine what they should or should not do as a general rule.

3.) *Applied Ethics*: Concerns what a person is obligated or permitted to do in a specific situation or a particular domain of action. In other words, it is the study of particular situations and the correct action(s) to take in those specific circumstances.[84]

You might notice that the concept of metaethics pertains directly to what you have done throughout this chapter. You have decided upon the very nature of morality/ethics itself; namely, whether it is objective or subjective, its source, and its purpose. This will help to inform your normative ethics by establishing a moral foundation that helps you determine what is right and wrong and what you generally should or should not do.

Your normative ethics can then be *applied* to certain situations to determine what the right course of action is under specific circumstances that you will encounter in your life. It is these latter two conceptions of ethics (normative and applied) that will be used to help you design a purposeful roadmap for your future in the next chapter. For now, let us consolidate your metaethical system by including it into your Foundational Document.

Chapter 7 Reflection Questions

1.) In your opinion, is morality objective or subjective in nature?

2.) What does your opinion on morality indicate about the *source* of morality?

3.) What does your opinion on morality indicate about the *purpose* of morality?

4.) Does your current understanding of morality conflict in any way from the moral system you lived by/were taught when you were younger? If so, how can you reconcile the two understandings?

8

Who You *Will* Be... and Why

Bringing it All Together

Thus far, we have taken a long journey toward discovering your sense of meaning and purpose. When learning any new concept or skill, it is important to take a break every now and then to briefly review what you have learned. This allows you to reconsolidate a solid foundation of context that you can then build new knowledge upon.

As a brief recap, we first explored the history of human meaning leading up to the current crisis that the Western world is facing. Following this, we looked at the five central reasons *why* this crisis of meaning has occurred. In Chapter 3, we looked at the standard and contextual definitions of 'meaning' and 'purpose' as well as useful conceptions of the two terms in order to help you establish your own definition of these terms and figure out what exactly it is you are searching for and/or are in need of. Following this, Chapter 4 explained the importance of self-awareness and Chapter 5 capitalized on this by allowing you to pursue your own self-discovery through examining your influences (both conscious and unconscious) and life factors (both positive and negative). Chapter 6 discussed the importance of a foundational core philosophy when searching for meaning and purpose, and Chapter 7 built upon this by discussing the nature of moral and ethical systems.

If you will notice, much of what we have done until this point has been retrospective in nature; that is, it has looked back towards what *once was* and what *has been*. In this chapter, we are going to look *forward* towards your future. As we discussed earlier, our sense of purpose, at its essence, not only gives us reason to continue moving forward towards the future, but also gives us reason to move toward the future *in a particular way*. Setting up how we wish the future to look like for ourselves, why we wish for it to look that way, and how we wish to achieve the goal of becoming our ideal self (despite the inevitable prospect of enduring some suffering along the way) naturally instills us with this much-needed sense of purpose and direction.

In other words, creating a roadmap for your life gives you something to keep striving for even though you will encounter obstacles along the way. The stronger your purpose, the more capable and willing you will be to meet these obstacles and push past them towards your goals. Planning towards your future helps to determine exactly what you are going to do in order to fulfill your purpose, thereby serving as a foundation for your journey from the present to the future. This is precisely why those who feel that they have no purpose in this life tend to seek immediate pleasures and are only concerned with their comfort in the present moment. With that being said, let us avoid this all-too-familiar tendency by observing the first necessary element in our roadmap to the future.

Your Morals and Core Values

When looking ahead to your future, it is important to consider all of the paths that are available to you. This can of course be rather intimidating, since the options available to you are nearly infinite. However, establishing a moral system and a series of values can help immensely by cutting down the number of options that are available to you. To give an exaggerated example, becoming a teacher might be in accordance with your morals and therefore a viable option, while becoming a drug dealer is likely to be decidedly less so. Evidently, this is not to say that this process effectively limits you in any negative way. Instead, it merely ensures that you are only investing your valuable time and effort in considering (and subsequently pursuing) life paths that will prove to be truly beneficial for you and those around you.

There is a valuable distinction to be made between morals and values, however. Whereas morals are rules that govern one's conduct, values are instead qualities that have intrinsic worth to us (and are therefore *determined* by our moral system). For example, if I believe that I have a moral obligation to take care of myself and strive to be the best I can be since I was fortunate enough to be granted the gift of life (whether by chance or by a creator), my corresponding value might be something like that of 'self-improvement' or 'personal development'.

It is certainly the case that many values can also be held *unconsciously* if we do not actively take the time to consider them. For instance, whatever you willingly choose to do at any given moment is reflective of what you value *at that given moment*. If I am sitting at my desk eating a peanut butter sandwich and contemplating life, I have likely subsconsciously made the decision that the action of doing so is my preferred action over any other option available, and therefore it is what I value most at that moment. Similarly, right now you are spending your time reading this book, which means you consciously or subconsciously value doing so over any other alternative at this present moment (and believe me, I am quite humbled!) You have likely made a subconscious decision that the value you will receive from this book is greater than that of scrolling through Twitter for hours on end, for example.

It is also worthy to note that many values *can* (and often *do*) conflict with one another. If my moral system involves living in a way that fosters self-improvement, then having some fun and getting adequate rest also have to be taken into account as essential values of mine. Too much of these activities, however, and they will inevitably work against my value of self-improvement (just like how *overworking* would harm my health despite probably bringing be closer to fulfilling other values of mine, at first). It is precisely reasons like these that demonstrate the need for ordering and prioritizing your values. Each one of your values inevitably has a different level of worth and importance as per the unique entailments of your moral system.

Life coach Tony Robbins formulated a fantastic exercise that pertains to these concepts and helps one to prioritize their values. Tony lists ten potential values and asks readers to rank-order them from most important to least important (numbered 1 through 10) in order to establish their own *hierarchy of values*. Briefly, and just in your head, take a moment to think about how you might order the following values in terms of their personal importance to you as an individual:

Love

Success

Freedom

Intimacy

Security

Adventure

Power

Passion

Comfort

Health[85]

You may notice at the outset that you have a strict preference for some of these values over others, and that is exactly the point that I am touching on here. Your moral system (that which provides guidelines and boundaries surrounding the actions you take and the behaviors you engage in) determines the things that you value (those things which have intrinsic worth and help to determine what is worthy of pursuing/attaining in your life and in what order).

Just as there are values that we wish to move toward, there are also things that we value moving *away from*. Take a look at these negative values and try to briefly rank-order them from most important to stay away from to least important to stay away from (numbered 1 through 8):

Rejection

Anger

Frustration

Loneliness

Depression

Failure

Humiliation

Guilt[86]

Quite an interesting thing to note is the fact that knowing what feelings you wish you stay *away from* actually helps to indicate in which direction you *should go* as well. Our moral system naturally takes both of these options into account by opening up paths that we believe we should go down and paths that we believe we should stay away from. While our moral system's entailments can leave numerous paths open to us, our values further specify which paths we most prioritize taking. Therefore, they work in conjunction with one another to establish purpose (a *reason* to move towards the future *in a particular way*).

It is also important to note that values *can* change. One of the most common examples is when someone gives birth to a child. Typically, their values tend to shift towards prioritizing love and providing comfort for that child, whereas occupational success might have once been their highest priority value prior to their child being born. You might even be able to remember various points in your life in which you yourself held different values (or had a different prioritization of certain values). While values can be established as a response to a certain event (such as having children), values can also be pre-emptively *created* and purposefully prioritized order to serve a desired purpose.

The extent to which you adhere to your values can be monitored simply by observing your regular actions. As such, at the end of this chapter you will be asked to indicate not only what values you currently hold (both consciously and unconsciously) by observing how you act, but also what values you *will need to have* in order to live your ideal life and achieve your life vision; your *ideal* values, in other words.

Your Responsibilities

In the Western world, especially within the past fifty years or so, we have seen a dramatic and seemingly exponential rise both in the extent to which individual rights and freedoms exist and the extent to which they are defended. These rights and freedoms are most often codified in the form of constitutional and/or statutory documents that enumerate a given set of rights and freedoms that citizens of a given country (or region) have.

Examples of these include the Canadian Charter of Rights and Freedoms and the U.S. Bill of Rights.

Following the creation of constitutional documents like these, the listed rights and freedoms that are enshrined within them are often later interpreted by the highest judiciary in the country. This usually occurs upon the emergence of a court case pertaining to the perceived violation of a citizens' rights. This process can lead to additional entailments that are *read into* the document's provisions or even mounting public pressure to make amendments to the document as a whole. As Western civilization has evolved and increasingly become more tolerant of different views and actions, the number of rights and freedoms that are recognized has increased quite proportionally.

As a general rule, rights and freedoms have the effect of advancing the human condition within the societies that they are instituted and are therefore a positive force. Of course, the possibility that they can extend too far is always there, such as the implementation of a right to hurt others, as a silly but quite illustrative hypothetical example. The advancement of rights and freedoms can also have unintended consequences, especially among those who were not granted them while they were living, but rather were born into a world in which those rights and freedoms pre-date them. The problem here is not inherent in the rights and freedoms themselves, but instead it is of these individuals' *conceptions* of them.

A poor conception of rights and freedoms might make one believe that they are in a sense untouchable and entitled to things from others; in other words, that others have a series of *responsibilities* towards them with no need for reciprocity on their behalf. As per these constitutional documents, in a sense they are partially correct about this last notion. These documents *do* indeed outline a series of rights and freedoms that citizens have (particularly in relation to their government). By virtue of the government being constitutionally bound to adhere to these enumerated rights and freedoms, the government, in effect, has *responsibility* for doing so.

Interestingly, there are two types of responsibility that the government must fulfill: *positive* responsibility (a responsibility to *grant* something to individuals, such as ensuring the safety and security of the individual as per their right to life and security) and *negative* responsibility (a responsibility *not* to infringe upon something that is perceived to be inherent to the individual, such as imprisoning them without just cause, which would infringe upon their right to a fair trial).

With all these rights and freedoms granted to them, people might consciously or unconsciously feel a sense of entitlement without firmly establishing their *own* responsibilities to others. The only legally codified responsibilities of the individual in most Western countries are to be found in criminal laws or bureaucratic regulations. Notice what these all have in common, however: they are laws or regulations dictating what an individual must *avoid* doing (do not kill others, do not steal from others, do not take up two or more parking spots with your oversized pick-up truck, etc.) Interestingly, these are all *negative* responsibilities. Positive responsibilities among citizens are not to be found in the laws of most Western countries.

Unfortunately enough, this fact leads those in Western society to perceive the term 'responsibility' as having a negative connotation when entrusted upon an individual. However, it is important to note that this negative connotation mostly arises from a negative mindset regarding the responsibilities that *others* impose upon *us*, which often makes us feel accountable to others instead of living our own life in the way that we want to. To illustrate this concept further, think of instances such as having to attend class when we do not want to or having to clean the house before our partner gets home. A simple shift in mindset toward qualifying these actions as responsibilities that *we* impose upon *ourselves* makes them much more tolerable (and often more exciting to fulfill, in fact).

This view is aptly described by author Mark Manson when he writes: "The more we choose to accept responsibility in our lives, the more power we will exercise over our lives. Accepting responsibility for our problems is thus the first step to solving them...A lot of people hesitate to take responsibility for their problems because they believe that to be *responsible* for your problems is to be *at fault* for your problems."[87] Perhaps because of the entitlement culture mentioned earlier, this 'fault and responsibility' conception also extends to the reverse situation; that is, when considering the responsibilities that others have towards us.

Manson goes on to write "There's a difference between blaming someone else for your situation and that person's [*sic*] actually being responsible for your situation. Nobody else is ever *responsible* for your situation but you. Many people may be to blame for your unhappiness, but nobody is ever responsible for your unhappiness but you. This is because *you* always get to choose how you see things, how you react to things, how you value things. You always get to choose the metric by which to measure your experiences."[88] If your partner were to cheat on you, for instance, yes it could be construed as being his/her *fault* that you are unhappy, but it is your *responsibility* to deal with the situation because no one else is on the receiving end of the treatment but you. You are you. It is a harsh truth, but a necessary one if you are to live a truly happy life. You are not in control of what other people do. Similarly, they should not be in control of what you do.

This shift in perception allows us to view these responsibilities as positive things that we *ourselves* have consciously determined will make our lives and the lives of others better. Instead of saying "Oh, my stupid professor is making me attend class every day", one might instead think "I have a responsibility to myself to attend class so that I do not stress myself out by missing important material that will be on the exam. I have also invested so much into my education that skipping class could jeopardize all of my expended time and effort. I have a responsibility to myself to become as knowledgeable as possible and succeed in these classes so that I can use that knowledge in my future career, which will make the world a better place and will make my life more meaningful."

Blaming others for the problems that you face constitutes an extraordinarily tempting yet harmful way of thinking and is indicative of a fixed mindset regarding your own capabilities. People often underestimate the extent to which they are capable of changing their lives and their mindsets. Yes, your circumstances can be (and often are) far from ideal, but it is precisely your mindset surrounding your circumstances and how you adapt to them that determines not only your character, but your sense of fulfillment in life. There are two primary options here: either perceive yourself as being a victim to outside circumstances and feel as though your life is entirely subject to the wishes others, or recognize, establish and fulfill the responsibilities that you personally create for yourself. The latter option is precisely what breeds confidence and a solidified sense of purpose in an individual.

This dichotomy highlights the importance of establishing your own positive responsibilities (both to yourself and others) that are necessitated by your own personal moral system and values. Too many people fail to consider the question "What do my moral system and values indicate that I should be doing for myself and for others?" Sure, you can have a moral system and values, but if you do not *act* upon them, if they are never *materialized*, they are essentially *worthless*. Having a purpose entails the *responsibility* of fulfilling that purpose. Having a moral code entails the *responsibility* of following that code and not acting outside of it when making decisions. Similarly, having values entails the *responsibility* of pursuing the things that you value in their order of priority/significance while operating within your moral code.

The key to an individual's sense of purpose, then, is the adoption and subsequent fulfillment of their moral responsibilities.

Try to think about this in a more practical and tangible way; let us imagine you are a college/university student (which you very well might be!) If you were to wake up at 1 p.m., sit down to play video games for 6 hours, then go out to the club to drink until 3 a.m., do you think you would feel truly happy and a deep sense of fulfillment? How about this, instead: imagine a day in which you woke up early to go for an outdoor jog, completed all of your homework, ate healthy, and called your parents to say hello and tell them that you miss them. While not as immediately pleasurable as playing video games or partying, would you not feel a deeper sense of happiness and fulfillment afterward? These feelings stem from fulfilling what you perceive to be your positive responsibilities (which, in this case, might be taking care of your health, educating yourself and setting yourself up well for your future, and contributing to the happiness of your parents).

The importance of aligning your responsibilities with your moral system cannot be overstated. Having responsibilities that are firmly rooted in your deepest moral convictions is the strongest way to ensure that they will be fulfilled. A sense of moral duty can be so powerful that it can even thwart our extraordinarily powerful instincts to survive. Suicide bombers, for instance, have such a strong (albeit very flawed) sense of moral duty that they are willing to kill themselves and others to fulfill what they unfortunately believe to be their moral responsibility.

On the complete opposite end of the moral spectrum, soldiers and police officers put their lives on the line daily out of a sense of moral duty to protect and serve their fellow citizens and their country. Grounding your responsibilities in your moral system is a crucial step in ensuring that they are not only legitimate in nature, but also that you believe in them and are willing to pursue them wholeheartedly.

In this chapter's reflection questions, we will outline the positive responsibilities that you have to yourself and others in your life as per the moral and value systems that you established in the previous chapter. It is my guess that you might be surprised as to how clear this makes the path ahead of you.

Your Ambitions and Goals

The importance of establishing your own goals and ambitions is perhaps no better illustrated than by one of the greatest athletes of all time. In 2008 at the Beijing Summer Olympic Games, the legendary swimmer Michael Phelps did the unthinkable and collected eight gold medals in a single Games while setting seven world records in the process. This eclipsed the former record of seven gold medals held by Mark Spitz from the 1972 Summer

Olympics in Munich, West Germany, making Phelps the most successful athlete ever at a single Olympics.

During the Beijing Olympics, Phelps also became the most decorated Olympian of *all time* in terms of gold medals, with his total of fourteen gold medals across two Olympics surpassing the previous record of nine. Even though he would successfully compete at two more Olympics following 2008, by this point he had already arguably become the most successful athlete of all time in terms of his capacity to achieve specifically planned (and seemingly unattainable) goals.[89]

Leading into the 2012 London Olympic Games, however, Phelps suffered from a lack of motivation and would frequently miss practices (and self-admittedly put little effort into the practices that he *did* attend). Looking back, he has noted that relative to Beijing 2008 his preparation for London 2012 was quite terrible.[90] In 2008 he had achieved almost everything there was that he could possibly achieve. As such, eclipsing what he was able to do in those Olympics would be, quite frankly, inconceivable and plainly unrealistic. In fact, Phelps pre-emptively precluded the possibility of even being able to do so by only entering in seven events for the London Games (as opposed to the eight that he had entered in for Beijing).[91]

With regard to his actual timed records, given his lack of preparation, older age, and the fact that the governing body for swimming (FINA) had changed the rules surrounding the swimsuits that swimmers were allowed to wear (making only slower-material suits available), it was extraordinarily unlikely that he would even be able to beat any of his best times in any event.

Evidently, the only conceivable goals that Phelps realistically had at this point would be to merely advance his legacy and beat the all-time Olympic record for the total number of medals won by an individual (no matter the color; gold, silver, or bronze). To do this, Phelps would only need two more medals of any color. Out of his seven events, he managed to get 4 gold medals and 2 silver medals for a total of six, a performance that he was very disappointed with. Following the London Olympics, Phelps retired from the sport of swimming, and later described his attitude following the decision as follows: "Done. Bye. See ya. Finished. Nothing… I wanted nothing to do with the sport. I was done…"[92]

Retirement brought about a sense of freedom that the previously hyper-dedicated and determined Michael Phelps had never known. He had all of the money and fame that he needed to live life to the worst. He gained thirty pounds, partied, drank, and in his words, "…had fun, probably too much fun." With swimming out of his life, he had no purpose and no direction; everything he had rooted his meaning and purpose in had ended and he had shunned it in resentment. He had no goals, no ambitions, and nothing to work towards besides exercising his freedom in every way possible. Eventually, in late 2014, Phelps hit rock bottom after getting charged with a DUI, with a blood alcohol level twice that of the legal limit.[93]

Following this, Phelps fell into a deep depression and contemplated suicide, prompting a stay in a behavioral rehabilitation facility. It was at this facility through his self-reflection and use of the resources available to him that Phelps would re-discover the meaning of his life and his purpose: "It has turned me into believing that there is a power greater than myself, and that there is a purpose for me on this planet." While Phelps has otherwise kept his moral and philosophical systems quite private, the events following this revelation make it relatively easy to discern some of his values, perceived responsibilities, and goals.[94]

Shortly after this turning point, Phelps got engaged to his fiancée and had a child, both of whom provided him with new responsibilities and an even deeper sense of purpose.[95] Phelps carried his newfound meaning and purpose into his unexpected comeback at the 2016 Rio Olympics, which his wife and newborn baby both attended. He went on to win 5 gold medals and one silver medal at the age of 31, which is strikingly old for a swimmer to win medals and was especially impressive given how out of shape he had been just over one year prior. Phelps was visibly emotional after almost every single one of his podium appearances and was much more expressive than he had been in the past. Typically, he had previously preferred to bottle his emotions up to maintain the image of perfection that the media had established for him.[96]

Phelps' story demonstrates the power of ambitions and goals in contributing to our sense of meaning and purpose. When Phelps' ambitions and goals were at their clearest, he was at his happiest and performed at his best. Phelps' story also helps to elucidate the difference between ambitions and goals in the first place. Anyone familiar with Phelps' story knows that his ambitions had always been to: change the sport of swimming (through garnering the respect that it deserves and making it more popular), to inspire others, and to save lives through encouraging water safety. These ambitions evidently stemmed from his perceived responsibilities, which were rooted in his values and moral system.

You might notice that his ambitions are quite broad; that is, there is no singular way to achieve them and they are not very specific. This is where his *goals* came in. For Phelps, his ambitions of changing the sport of swimming and inspiring others were achieved by achieving *goals* that no one had ever done before, such as breaking a certain number of world records, getting a certain number of medals, getting a certain time in a particular event, etc., which would inevitably draw attention to the sport. His ambition of encouraging water safety was achieved through his goal of setting up a foundation dedicated to teaching kids how to swim and lead healthier lives.[97] Eventually, the circumstances in the lowest part of his life encouraged him to establish the ambition of promoting mental health awareness, which he achieved through his goals of joining the board of a mental health organization and speaking out more openly and publicly about his own struggles (which he had never done in the past).[98]

As can be seen in the example of Michael Phelps, goals serve as specific ways in which one's broader ambitions can be achieved. If my broader ambitions are to educate people and improve their lives, for instance, I might have more specific goals of writing a self-help book and establishing a multimedia platform dedicated to achieving those ambitions. Since your ambitions are rooted in your perceived responsibilities as per your established moral and value systems, it might be helpful to establish an overall *life mission statement* from which your ambitions can originate. This statement can be as short as one sentence, and should be reflective of what you wish your overall legacy to be on Earth.

Goals themselves also require a lot of work to achieve, of course. Phelps achieved his goals by systematically training day in and day out, ensuring he had proper rest and nutrition, etc. Goals that collectively lead toward the fulfillment of an ambition are best achieved by forming a habitual *roadmap* or plan toward their achievement.

Your Purpose-Driven Roadmap

Now that you have a better understanding of the interrelationship between ambitions and goals, it is important to understand exactly how one can design a roadmap toward their achievement. The creation of a roadmap toward achieving one's ambitions and goals will naturally be unique to each and every individual. Michael Phelps' roadmap creation process, for instance, involved writing down the goal times he wished to achieve and planning out how he could achieve them with his coach, Bob Bowman. Despite the differentiation in the roadmap creation process among individuals, there are two key components that apply to everyone when creating theirs: *habits* and *major actions*.

Habits refer to micro-actions that are done regularly, and usually on a daily basis. Habits allow an individual to set their lifestyle and health up in an ideal manner so that they can successfully and effectively conduct major actions, which lead to the achievement of goals and ambitions. Any goal or ambition is likely to be something that is relatively challenging for you to achieve (otherwise, they would be ordinary occurrences and therefore not meaningful nor especially significant).

As such, the successful achievement of a given goal or ambition is accomplished through the pursuit of challenging major actions, which are made possible by you functioning at your best. In turn, functioning at your best obviously requires healthy and productive daily habits. The methods that allow you to achieve your ambitions and goals, habits included, should all be nested within your overarching moral responsibilities.

As we observed in Chapter 5, you currently have both good habits and bad habits that you engage in. Your good habits are likely to help you achieve your ambitions, while your bad habits are those that inhibit your ability to achieve them. Consequently, successfully conducting your major actions towards your goals requires four key habit commitments:

(1) Maintaining the good habits you currently engage in.

(2) Seeking to engage in good habits that you *a.)* do not currently engage in and/or *b.)* are not currently aware of. These constitute part of a vital ongoing learning process about your health and well-being.

(3) Ceasing the bad habits that you currently engage in.

(4) Further analyzing and reflecting upon your current habits, some of which you might not know are bad for you. Again, this is categorized under ongoing learning about what is good or bad for you.

Major actions, on the other hand, are larger actions that more overtly move you closer toward the achievement of your goals. For Michael Phelps, for instance, his habits might have included getting enough sleep each night and maintaining a healthy diet, but a major action would be something like going to a local swim meet to measure his progress on the way to a bigger international competition. Major actions then, are sequential in nature; that is, they build upon one another in the direction of your goal and bring you closer and closer in steps. For this reason, it is extremely helpful to write out your roadmap as a series of steps that logically and chronologically follow one another and ultimately lead to the achievement of your goals and ambitions.

When establishing your responsibilities, ambitions, goals, etc., it is important to remember to operate within your sphere of influence, just as you did when acknowledging your major failures in Chapter 5. Feeling that you are responsible for the well-being of every single human being on Earth is of course unreasonable, just like the ambition to single-handedly solve world poverty.

Beginning with the responsibility of advancing the well-being of the people in your family and friend groups is a good start, and looking to solve poverty in your local community would be a more reasonable initial ambition (after all, who knows where one can go from there!)

Do not hold yourself responsible for things that you cannot control since this will only lead to hurt. With that being said, be sure not to limit yourself. It is best to begin with the things that you know you are reasonably responsible for and increase the scope of this responsibility only when you are able. This way, you are not placing limits on yourself, but rather are taking small steps initially to avoid overreaching at the outset.

In today's capitalist society there are further limitations with regards to the ambitions that you can have since, of course, you must be able to financially support yourself and/or your family in the process. This typically requires having an occupation that consists of forty hours of your time per week, not including the time it takes for transportation and other preparation. Since a large majority of your time and effort will be put towards this job, it is important that your occupation is commensurate with your sense of purpose and your biggest ambitions; that is, you can fulfill them through the proper fulfillment of your job so that you can support yourself financially at the same time. Often, money serves as a *means* to achieve values (such as supporting your family), but it should not be construed as a value *in and of itself.*

Having an unfulfilling career is another major detriment to many peoples' sense of meaning and purpose. In having such a career, they are not pursuing their true ambitions and as such do not feel a sense of moral fulfillment. What I would highly recommend is reflecting back upon your foundational document once it is finished, and looking at your skills, traits, areas of specialty, moral system, values, responsibilities, ambitions, and goals and aligning these with a suitable career in which you can employ the use of your greatest skills in order to fulfill your moral responsibilities and ambitions.

This is definitely easier said than done for those who are already engaged in a long-time career that they dislike and/or are financially unable to find something else to pursue at the moment. However, if this is indeed the case, now that you have a better idea of what you are seeking you can try to implement these things and act upon your purpose *within* your current job; you might be surprised with the results if you take the initiative and pursue creative methods to do so. Just as we are able to maintain and act upon our own individual moral system within the confines a society that has a collective moral foundation, so too can you act towards your moral purpose within most occupations that are out there; you just have to know where your skills and capabilities can be utilized.

The same notion applies to those of you who are students, as well. Ensure that your major concentration, areas of speciality, and chosen classes not only align with your skillset, but also that you know how you wish to use them to fulfill your purpose in the future. This will help to also naturally cultivate a deep interest in your education at the same time, which almost always leads to further success. Whether it is high school or college/university, education is of course an investment for the future, but that does not mean that you are unable to start fulfilling your purpose while you pursue it.

If you begin to learn how to foster your well-being, good habits, and act upon the entailments of your foundational document both in school and in other extracurricular activities, you will reap exceptional and exponential benefits once you are out into the 'real world'. Post-secondary school is most often the place where young adults begin to feel the drain of nihilism and a lack of moral standards, but rest assured that those who earn the most respect and admiration (and those who are the happiest) are not those who party the hardest for four years, but instead are those who emerge from their education with a sense of purpose, a plan, and an actualized desire for health, happiness, and success.

Chapter 8 Reflection Questions

Values

1.) Reflect upon what you currently spend your time doing and how your time is divided on a daily/weekly basis. What does this indicate about the things that you value? Be honest with yourself!

2.) What sorts of values would you need to have in order to live what you would consider to be an ideal life?

Responsibilities

3.) What responsibilities do you have to *yourself* and to *others* (your family, partner, friends, community, the world, mentors, etc.)? Create a unique list of responsibilities for each relevant group.

Ambitions, Goals, Major Actions, and Habits

4.) Come up with a brief overall mission statement for your life. What do you want your legacy to be? How would you like people do describe your life and your impact once you are gone?

5.) What are some of your broader ambitions in life that pertain to your overall mission? Remember to align them with your responsibilities!

6.) What goals will you need to accomplish in order to fulfill each ambition?

7.) Create a sequential roadmap (a list of numbered steps or major actions) that demonstrates how you will achieve your goals and ambitions.

8.) What daily habits would set your life up in a way that would make it the most ideal in order to accomplish your goals and take major actions? Try to outline an ideal day.

The Schillerian Model of Meaning & Purpose

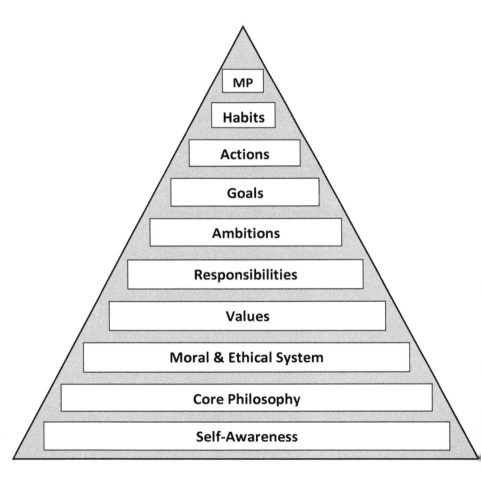

Life, Revisited

By now the above model is likely to make much more sense to you than it did at the start of this book. In creating your Foundational Document, you progressed step-by-step through this model in order to establish a clearer understanding of your own sense of meaning and purpose in the life that you are currently living. As we near the end of this journey, it is important to tie everything that you have learned together to see how all the elements of this model work together to provide a foundation for living a meaningful and purposeful life.

When used in tandem as a sequential process, these components of life are a fascinating and powerful force that can truly change lives for the better as I am sure they will do for you. If it helps you to better conceptualize the model, you can also think of it as an *equation* – adding up, understanding, and implementing the value of all of these components will help you to find the answers that you are looking for; namely, a clearer sense of meaning and purpose in your life. As our journey draws to a close, let us look more closely at how these components relate to (and work with) one another to form an integrated whole.

(I) Self-Awareness

This component of the model refers to the observation of your own thought patterns and behaviors, and the subsequent taking of action upon those observations. This includes observing things like **Unconscious Influences** (Sociocultural, Familial, and Sociodemographic), **Conscious Influences** (External, Educational, and Biological/Psychological), **Positive Life Factors** (Accomplishments, Good Traits, Skills, Areas of Specialty, and Good Habits), and **Negative Life Factors** (Failures, Bad Traits, Lacking Skills, Areas for Improvement, and Bad Habits).

Understanding these influences and factors allows you to be more aware of yourself and any potential biases you may have while operating in life. Furthermore, discerning what you perceive to be good and bad about your life allows you to get a foundational understanding of what you value and also summarizes the way in which you have experienced life and how those experiences have shaped you. Once you know yourself, you are then able to more accurately know the things that are outside of you. This permits you to more thoroughly establish and assess your own **Core Philosophy** in an unbiased and unrestricted manner.

(II) Core Philosophy

Your core philosophy refers to your core belief system about the fundamental nature of reality and existence, most importantly referring to the *origins* of your existence. Our thoughts about how the universe began can be informed not only by our unconscious influences, but also by our conscious reflections using the systems of rational thought that we develop as we grow older. Your core philosophy determines whether you believe the universe (and by extension, you as an individual) was created purposefully, or if it happened by chance.

There are three fundamental positions that one can take with regard to this question: **Theism**, **Atheism**, or **Agnosticism**. While all three are viable options in establishing a sense of meaning or significance with regard to your existence, they each impact the course of one's life substantially and in varying ways. Your core philosophy directly determines the fundamental nature and source of your **Moral & Ethical System**.

(III) Moral & Ethical System

Your moral and ethical system refers to both your intuitive and reasoned notions surrounding how you should act throughout your life. It serves as a guideline that governs your actions and creates a more streamlined vision for your future by justifiably eliminating many of the options available to you (namely, those that are considered to be morally unacceptable). Your moral and ethical system can be based in either an Objective (created by a god or gods) or Subjective (created by humanity) view of morality. No matter which view you adhere to, your sense of morality and ethics will help determine the **Values** that you aspire to.

(IV) Values

While your moral system provides rules/guidelines that broadly governs our conduct, our values are qualities that have intrinsic worth to us (whether they are qualities of ourselves such as intelligence, or general qualities of interpersonal relations such as humility, honesty, love, and friendship). Establishing a **Hierarchy of Values** allows us to further prioritize which path we should take in the future, working in tandem with our moral system to create both a clearer vision of the future and a clearer purpose to work towards. Knowing the things that we value allows us to form time-specific **Responsibilities**.

(V) Responsibilities

This component of the model merely refers to the things that you are required to do as per your own moral system and values. It is immensely important to consider not only the rules that govern our conduct (i.e. what we should *not* do) and in what ways our values are prioritized, but also what these two things dictate that we *should* do. An individual has numerous responsibilities in life, but it is pre-eminently important to take the proper time to consider purpose-driven responsibilities to yourself and those around you. The challenge of fulfilling of your responsibilities necessarily gives you a purpose to strive towards. Without responsibilities, we would be moving from the present to the future feeling that there is nothing that we *ought* to do, and would therefore lack a *purpose* moving forward. Our responsibilities are both fulfilled by and reflected in our **Ambitions, Goals, Major Actions, and Habits**.

(VI) Ambitions, Goals, Major Actions, and Habits

Ambitions are broader things that we wish to achieve over an extended period of time, and are informed by our responsibilities. **Goals** are a series of desired sequential results (achieved through the investment of time and effort) that, if they are all accomplished, will achieve the effect of fulfilling our broader ambition(s). **Major Actions**

are significant steps that we take toward achieving our goals. **Habits** are regular (and usually daily) practices that set our life up in a manner that is ideal for us conduct major actions to achieve our goals, typically through advancing the status of our mental and physical well-being.

Putting it Into Practice

If in the future you ever need a reminder as to the process through which you established your meaning and purpose, the above section is here for quick reference. I highly suggest that you organize, polish, and review your Foundational Document as much as you possibly can. Since creating my own, I have found it so immensely important to my everyday life that I have carried it around with me almost anywhere I go, as have several of my clients. Having it to reflect upon and remind myself of my own self-created purpose and where I hope to be in the future has been absolutely invaluable and extremely motivating. Whenever you are feeling down or unmotivated, it is extraordinarily useful to look back upon that which you have carefully created and that which defines everything about who you have been, currently are, and will be.

Over the next week, challenge yourself to live according to your meaning and purpose by starting to institute the entailments of your Foundational Document into your life. Think of your Foundational Document as a personalized contract that you have made with yourself – one that you *know* will undeniably make your life better since you thought it to be worth creating *and* put so much care into creating it in order to help yourself. With the work that you have put into creating it and all of the things that you have learned throughout this book, I have no doubt that you will have found the motivation to strive towards your ideal self by fostering your own well-being and that of those around you.

Following the entailments of something like this out of our own accord can be extremely compelling and rewarding. Never forget that when we live in accordance with our meaning and purpose is when we are truly happy and are able to help others reach that same true happiness instead of endlessly chasing immediate pleasure. Venture out into the world with the unshakeable confidence of not only knowing what you are truly here for and what you are here to do, but also having put the work in to find these things out for yourself, which very few people manage to do. One of the most incredible and inspiring things about life is that there is *always* room for improvement; as such, continue to learn and grow as you help others do the same. Your ideal self is out there in the realm of possibility - it is up to you and you alone to bring it to fruition.

Live your ideal life. Always.

About The Author

As a certified Canadian educator, author, and personal consultant, Luke Schiller aspires to improve the lives of people around the world. Having experienced the impact of his own self-improvement journey, he is inspired by the belief that dedication to the improvement of oneself in all areas of life has a transformative effect that inevitably diffuses outward to those around you and ultimately makes the world a better place.

Luke holds a Bachelor of Arts in History and Political Science (with an Emphasis in Law & Policy) from Trent University, a Bachelor of Education from Queen's University, and a Master of Arts in Political Science (with an Emphasis in Comparative Politics & International Relations) from Queen's University, during which he swam competitively for the Queen's University Varsity Swim Team.

Combining his vast interdisciplinary knowledge with his extensive pedagogical training, Luke strives to strike a much-needed balance between remaining informative yet practical in his written and audiovisual content. For more from Luke, be sure to visit his official website at **www.schilleracademy.com**

Notes

INTRODUCTION

[1] Max Roser, "War and Peace: Global Deaths in Conflicts Since 1400" https://www.ourworldindata.org/war-and-peace (accessed September 8th, 2018).

[2] Jean M. Twenge et al., "Birth Cohort Increases in Psychopathology Among Young Americans, 1938–2007: A Cross-Temporal Meta-Analysis of the MMPI," *Clinical Psychology Review vol. 30* (2010): 145-154.

[3] Jean M. Twenge, "Are Mental Health Issues on the Rise?" https://www.psychologytoday.com/ca/blog/our-changing-culture/201510/are-mental-health-issues-the-rise (accessed September 8th, 2018).

CHAPTER 1

[4] Chris Harman, *A People's History of the World: From the Stone Age to the New Millenium* (New York: Verso Books, 2008), 5.

[5] Ibid, 6.

[6] Ibid, 8-9.

[7] Robert Wright, *The Evolution of God* (New York: Little, Brown and Company, 2009), 17.

[8] Ibid, 17-19.

[9] Ted Honderich, ed., *The Oxford Companion to Philosophy* (Oxford: Oxford University Press, 1995), 666.

[10] Robert C. Solomon and Douglas McDermid, *Introducing Philosophy for Canadians* (Toronto: Oxford University Press, 2011), 2.

[11] Ibid, 2.

[12] John M. Cooper, ed., *Plato: Complete Works* (Indianapolis: Hackett Publishing Company, 1997), 23.

[13] Bryan Magee, *The Great Philosophers: An Introduction to Western Philosophy* (Oxford: Oxford University Press, 2000), 34.

[14] Brian M. Fagan and Charlotte Beck, ed., *The Oxford Companion to Archaeology* (Oxford: Oxford University Press, 1996), 762.

[15] Brent Nongbri, *Before Religion: A History of a Modern Concept* (New Haven: Yale University Press, 2013). The corresponding definition was constructed under the inspiration of the discussion in Part 1 of this work.

[16] Solomon and McDermid, 117.

[17] David P. Mindell, *The Evolving World: Evolution in Everyday Life* (Cambridge: Harvard University Press, 2006), 224.

[18] Solomon and McDermid, 117.

[19] Conrad Hackett et al., *The Global Religious Landscape: A Report on the Size and Distribution of the World's Major Religious Groups as of 2010* (Washington, D.C.: The Pew Research Forum on Religion & Public Life, 2012), 18.

[20] Ibid, 22.

[21] Conrad Hackett and David McClendon, "Christians Remain World's Largest Religious Group, but They Are Declining in Europe" http://www.pewresearch.org/fact-tank/2017/04/05/christians-remain-worlds-largest-religious-group-but-they-are-declining-in-europe/ (accessed September 10th, 2018).

[22] BBC Health, "De-coding the Black Death" http://news.bbc.co.uk/2/hi/health/1576875.stm (accessed September 10th, 2018).

[23] United Nations Population Division, *The World At Six Billion* (New York: United Nations Department of Economic and Social Affairs, 1999), 5.

[24] Donald A. Cress, trans., *René Descartes: Meditations on First Philosophy* (Indianapolis: Hackett Publishing Company, 1993).

[25] Andrew Heywood, *Global Politics* (New York: Palgrave Macmillan, 2011), 112.

CHAPTER 2

[26] John L.E. Dreyer, *History of Astronomy from Thales to Kepler* (Cambridge: Cambridge University Press, 1906), 343.

[27] Maurice A. Finocchiaro, *Defending Copernicus and Galileo: Critical Reasoning in the Two Affairs* (New York: Springer Publishing Company, 2010), 74.

[28] Christopher J. Conselice et al., "The Evolution Of Galaxy Number Density At Z < 8 and Its Implications" *The Astrophysical Journal* vol. 830(2) (2016): 10.

[29] NASA, "NASA's Hubble Shows Milky Way is Destined for Head-On Collision" https://www.nasa.gov/mission_pages/hubble/science/milky-way-collide.html (accessed September 16th, 2018).

[30] Philip Plait, *Death from the Skies* (New York: Viking Press, 2008), 259.

[31] K.-P. Shröder and Robert Connon Smith, "Distant Future of the Sun and Earth Revisited" *Monthly Notices of the Royal Astronomical Society* vol. 386(1) (2008): 155-163.

[32] National Academy of Sciences, *Science and Creationism: A View from the National Academy of Sciences* (Washington, D.C.: The National Academies Press, 1999), 4-5.

[33] Beverly Stearns and Steven Stearns, *Watching, from the Edge of Extinction* (New York: Yale University Press, 1999), Preface page X.

[34] Internet Encyclopedia of Philosophy, "The Logical Problem of Evil" https://www.iep.utm.edu/evil-log/#H1 (accessed September 11th, 2018).

[35] Conrad Hackett et al., *The Age Gap in Religion Around the World* (Washington, D.C.: The Pew Research Center, 2012), 18-19.

[36] David B. Barrett and Todd M. Johnson, "Annual Statistical Table on World Religions, 1900-2025" http://www.wnrf.org/cms/statuswr.shtml (accessed September 11th, 2018).

[37] Conrad Hackett et al., *The Global Religious Landscape*, 24.

[38] Conrad Hackett et al., *The Future of World Religions: Population Growth Projections, 2010-2050* (Washington, D.C.: The Pew Research Center, 2015), 81.

[39] Ibid, 82.

[40] Gregory Smith et al., *America's Changing Religious Landscape* (Washington, D.C.: The Pew Research Center, 2015), 70.

[41] Conrad Hackett et al., *The Age Gap in Religion Around the World*, 64-67.

[42] Alison Flood, "Richard Dawkins to Give Away Copies of The God Delusion in Islamic Countries" https://www.theguardian.com/books/2018/mar/20/richard-dawkins-to-give-away-copies-of-the-god-delusion-in-islamic-countries (accessed September 12th, 2018).

[43] Josh Timonen, "The God Delusion One-Year Countdown" https://web.archive.org/web/20080828171533/http://richarddawkins.net/article,1599,The-God-Delusion-One-Year-Countdown,RichardDawkinsnet (accessed September 12th, 2018).

[44] Youtube, "Search Results of the Term 'Richard Dawkins' Sorted by Descending View Count" https://www.youtube.com/results?search_query=richard+dawkins&sp=CAM%253D (accessed August 29th, 2018).

[45] Youtube, "Search Results of the Term 'Christopher Hitchens' Sorted by Descending View Count" https://www.youtube.com/results?sp=CAM%253D&search_query=christopher+hitchens (accessed August 29th, 2018).

[46] Youtube, "Search Results of the Term 'Sam Harris' Sorted by Descending View Count" https://www.youtube.com/results?sp=CAM%253D&search_query=sam+harris (accessed August 29th, 2018).

[47] Statistica: The Statistics Portal, "Percentage of U.S. Internet Users Who Use YouTube as of January 2018, By Age Group" https://www.statista.com/statistics/296227/us-youtube-reach-age-gender/ (accessed September 12th, 2018).

[48] Robert L. Heilbroner, "The New Palgrave Dictionary of Economics" https://static1.squarespace.com/static/53ce7840e4b01d2bd01192ee/t/557f3b7ce4b09caf90c3c0f4/1434401660513/HeilbronerMilberg.pdf (accessed September 12th, 2018).

[49] John F. Helliwell et al., *World Happiness Report 2018* (New York: Sustainable Development Solutions Network, 2018), 20-22.

[50] National Center on Sexual Exploitation, "Pornography and Public Health Research Summary" http://www.endsexualexploitation.org/wp-content/uploads/NCOSE_Pornography-PublicHealth_ResearchSummary_8-2_17_FINAL-with-logo.pdf (accessed September 12th, 2018)

[51] R.E. Brown, "Sexual Arousal, the Coolidge Effect and Dominance in the Rat (*Rattus Norvegicus*)" *Animal Behaviour*, 22(3): 634–637.

[52] Your Brain on Porn (Website Name), "Studies Find Escalation and Habituation in Porn Users (Tolerance)" https://www.yourbrainonporn.com/studies-find-escalation-porn-users (accessed September 12th, 2018).

[53] National Center on Sexual Exploitation, "Pornography and Public Health Research Summary", 4-24.

CHAPTER 3

[54] Newton, Isaac. "Letter from Sir Isaac Newton to Robert Hooke" from the Historical Society of Pennsylvania https://discover.hsp.org/Record/dc-9792/Description (accessed October 28th, 2018).

[55] Merriam-Webster Dictionary, "Definition of *Meaning*" https://www.merriam-webster.com/dictionary/meaning (accessed September 12th, 2018).

[56] Richard Peacock, "The Probability of Life" http://www.evolutionfaq.com/articles/probability-life (accessed September 12th, 2018).

[57] Wikipedia, "Rare Earth Hypothesis" https://en.wikipedia.org/wiki/Rare_Earth_hypothesis (accessed September 12th, 2018.)

[58] Ibid.

[59] J. Schneider "Interactive Extra-solar Planets Catalog" *The Extrasolar Planets Encyclopedia* http://www.exoplanet.eu/catalog/ (accessed September 12th, 2018).

[60] Planetary Habitability Laboratory at the University of Puerto Rico at Arecibo, "Habitable Exoplanets Catalog" http://phl.upr.edu/projects/habitable-exoplanets-catalog (accessed September 12th, 2018).

[61] M. R. Rampino and S.H. Ambrose, (2000). "Volcanic Winter in the Garden of Eden: The Toba Supereruption and the Late Pleistocene Human Population Crash" *Special Paper of the Geological Society of America* vol. 345, 71-82.

[62] Carl Sagan, *Cosmos: A Personal Voyage, Episode 1* (Documentary Series: Public Broadcasting Service, 1990), 5:15 Timestamp.

[63] Oxford Dictionary, "Definition of *Purpose*" https://en.oxforddictionaries.com/definition/purpose (accessed September 12th, 2018).

[64] Jonathan Barnes, ed., *Nicomachean Ethics* from *The Complete Works of Aristotle* (Princeton: Princeton University Press, 1984).

[65] Jordan B. Peterson, *12 Rules For Life: An Antidote to Chaos* (Toronto: Random House Canada, 2018), 15.

[66] R. Ligneul and J.-C. Dreher, "Social Dominance Representations in the Human Brain" in *Decision Neuroscience: An Integrative Approach* (New York: Elsevier Inc., 2017), 211-214.

[67] Encyclopaedia Britannica, "Eudaemonism" https://www.britannica.com/topic/eudaemonism#ref273308 (accessed September 17th, 2018).

CHAPTER 4

[68] Joseph Luft and Harrington Ingham, "The Johari Window, A Graphic Model of Interpersonal Awareness" in *Proceedings of the Western Training Laboratory in Group Development* (Los Angeles: University of California, 1955).

[69] Tony Robbins, *Awaken the Giant Within* (New York: Simon & Schuster Paperbacks, 1991), 77.

[70] Ibid, 80.

[71] Carol Dweck, "Chapter 1: What Does This All Mean For You? The Two Mindsets" in *Mindset: The New Psychology of Success* (New York: Random House, 2006).

[72] Ibid.

CHAPTER 5

[73] Carl G. Jung et al., *Man and His Symbols* (New York: J.G. Ferguson Publishing, 1964) 26-31.

[74] Paul Reber, "What Is the Memory Capacity of the Human Brain?" *Scientific American* https://www.scientificamerican.com/article/what-is-the-memory-capacity/ (accessed September 12th, 2018).

CHAPTER 6

[75] Oxford Dictionary, "Definition of *Theism*" https://en.oxforddictionaries.com/definition/theism (accessed September 12th, 2018).

[76] Oxford Dictionary, "Definition of *Atheism*" https://en.oxforddictionaries.com/definition/atheism (accessed September 12th, 2018).

[77] Oxford Dictionary, "Definition of *Agnostic*" https://en.oxforddictionaries.com/definition/agnostic (accessed September 12th, 2018).

[78] Kayonda Hubert Ngamaba and Debbie, "Are Happiness and Life Satisfaction Different Across Religious Groups? Exploring Determinants of Happiness & Life Satisfaction" *Journal of Religion and Health*, 2017: 8.

CHAPTER 7

[79] James Rachels and Stuart Rachels, *The Elements of Moral Philosophy* (New York: McGraw-Hill, 2012), 13.

[80] Jordan B. Peterson, *Maps of Meaning* (New York: Routledge, 1999), 1.

[81] Colin Allen and Marc Bekoff, "Animal Play and the Evolution of Morality: An Ethological Approach" *Topoi* vol. 24, 2005, 125.

[82] Jordan B. Peterson, "Biblical Series III: God and the Hierarchy of Authority" https://www.youtube.com/watch?v=R_GPAI_q2QQ (accessed September 18th, 2018).

[83] Elisabeth Kübler-Ross and David Kessler, *On Grief & Grieving: Finding the Meaning of Grief Through the Five Stages of Loss* (New York: Scribner, 2014).

[84] All three definitions are derived from information available at: Internet Encyclopedia of Philosophy, "Ethics" https://www.iep.utm.edu/ethics/ (accessed October 8th, 2018).

CHAPTER 8

[85] Tony Robbins, *Awaken the Giant Within*, 349.

[86] Ibid, 356.

[87] Mark Manson, *The Subtle Art of Not Giving a F***: A Counterintuitive Approach to Living a Good Life* (New York: HarperOne, 2016), 96-97.

[88] Ibid, 99.

[89] CNN, "Phelps Wins Historic Eigth Gold Medal" http://www.edition.cnn.com/2008/SPORT/08/17/phelps.history.eight.g olds/ (accessed September 13th, 2018).

[90] Michael E. Ruane, "Testing the Limits" https://www.washingtonpost.com/sf/sports/wp/2016/06/09/testing-the-limits/?utm_term=.c7b383d7eaa4 (accessed September 13th, 2018).

[91] Alfie Crow, "2012 Olympics: Michael Phelps To Swim 7 Events In London" https://www.sbnation.com/london-olympics-2012/2012/7/2/3132063/michael-phelps-2012-olympics-london-seven-events (accessed September 13th, 2018).

[92] SportsCenter Featured "The Power of Sports: The Evolution of Michael Phelps" https://youtu.be/nnrMtFro-_w (accessed September 13th, 2018).

[93] Ibid.

[94] Ibid.

[95] Michael E. Ruane, "Testing the Limits".

[96] Chicago Tribune, "Golden finale: Michael Phelps Captures His 23rd Olympic Gold With Relay Win" http://www.chicagotribune.com/sports/international/ct-rio-olympics-mens-swimming-4x100m-medley-relay-20160813-story.html (accessed September 13th, 2018).

[97] Bob Considine, "Phelps to Use $1 Million Bonus to Start Charity" https://web.archive.org/web/20100728125731/http://today.msnbc.msn.com/id/26506320 (accessed September 13th, 2018).

[98] Medibio, "Board of Directors" http://medibio.com.au/board-of-directors/ (accessed September 13th, 2018).

CPSIA information can be obtained
at www.ICGtesting.com
Printed in the USA
LVHW112019091118
596620LV00001B/4/P